Yogic Management of
Asthma and Diabetes

Yogic Management of Asthma and Diabetes

Dr Swami Shankardevananda
MBBS (Sydney), MSc (UNSW)

Under the Guidance of
Swami Satyananda Saraswati

Yoga Publications Trust, Munger, Bihar, India

Printed by Bihar School of Yoga
    First published 1977
    Reprinted 1979, 1982
    Second edition 1986
    Reprinted 1993

Printed by Yoga Publications Trust
    Third edition 2002

ISBN: 81-85787-23-9
Price: Indian rupees one hundred only

Publisher and distributor: Yoga Publications Trust, Ganga Darshan, Munger, Bihar, India.

Website: www.yogavision.net
E-mail: ypt@yogavision.net

Printed at Thomson Press (India) Limited, New Delhi, 110001

SWAMI SIVANANDA SARASWATI

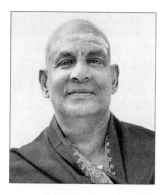

Swami Sivananda was born at Patta-madai, Tamil Nadu, in 1887. After serving as a medical doctor in Malaya, he renounced his practice, went to Rishikesh and was initiated into Dashnami sannyasa in 1924 by Swami Vishwananda Saraswati. He toured extensively throughout India, inspiring people to practise yoga and lead a divine life. He founded the Divine Life Society at Rishikesh in 1936, the Sivananda Ayurvedic Pharmacy in 1945, the Yoga Vedanta Forest Academy in 1948 and the Sivananda Eye Hospital in 1957. During his lifetime Swami Sivananda guided thousands of disciples and aspirants all over the world and authored over 200 books.

SWAMI SATYANANDA SARASWATI

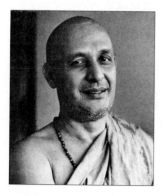

Swami Satyananda was born at Almora, Uttar Pradesh, in 1923. In 1943 he met Swami Sivananda in Rishikesh and adopted the Dashnami sannyasa way of life. In 1955 he left his guru's ashram to live as a wandering mendicant and later founded the International Yoga Fellowship in 1963 and the Bihar School of Yoga in 1964. Over the next 20 years Swami Satyananda toured internationally and authored over 80 books. In 1987 he founded Sivananda Math, a charitable institution for aiding rural development, and the Yoga Research Foundation. In 1988 he renounced his mission, adopting kshetra sannyasa, and now lives as a paramahamsa sannyasin.

SWAMI NIRANJANANANDA SARASWATI

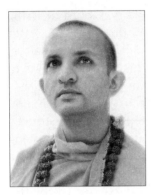

Swami Niranjanananda was born at Rajnandgaon, Madhya Pradesh, in 1960. At the age of four he joined the Bihar School of Yoga and was initiated into Dashnami sannyasa at the age of ten. From 1971 he travelled overseas and toured many countries for the next 11 years. In 1983 he was recalled to India and appointed President of Bihar School of Yoga. During the following 11 years he guided the development of Ganga Darshan, Sivananda Math and the Yoga Research Foundation. In 1990 he was initiated as a paramahamsa and in 1993 anointed preceptor in succession to Swami Satyananda. Bihar Yoga Bharati was founded under his direction in 1994. He has authored over 20 books and guides national and international yoga programs.

SWAMI SATYASANGANANDA SARASWATI

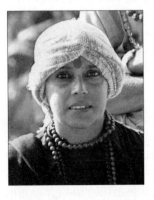

Swami Satyasangananda (Satsangi) was born on 24th March 1953, in Chandorenagore, West Bengal. From the age of 22 she experienced a series of inner awakenings which led her to her guru, Swami Satyananda. From 1981 she travelled ceaselessly with her guru in India and overseas and developed into a scholar with deep insight into the yogic and tantric traditions as well as modern sciences and philosophies. She is an efficient channel for the transmission of her guru's teachings. The establishment of Sivananda Math in Rikhia is her creation and mission, and she guides all its activities there, working tirelessly to uplift the weaker and underprivileged areas. She embodies compassion with clear reason and is the foundation of her guru's vision.

Contents

Research on Asthma and Diabetes

Appendices

Asthma and Yoga

1

Personal Reminiscences

What is the cause of asthma? This question has baffled western science up to this day. Therefore, we are presenting certain episodes from the author's early childhood experiences which we feel directly contributed to his disease. It is hoped that the reader may discover parallels in his own experiences. This account should be seen as the point of view of an ex-sufferer from asthma, who is now a medical doctor and a student of other branches of healing therapies.

Early beginnings

During my childhood, both of my parents were forced to work due to financial circumstances. It was necessary, as a result, to bring in a nurse as a surrogate mother to attend to my needs. Disagreement between us arose from the start on food, bedtime and many other things.

Out of many incidents, one experience in particular stands out in my mind. A disagreement involving food was resolved by my being force-fed, resulting in an attack of vomiting. I was unable to eat that particular food again for years. When, through yoga, I began to re-evaluate painful experiences, this episode came vividly to mind. As I relived the experience with a new understanding and equanimity, my dislike for this food was cured and the negative influence of the entire incident was erased.

There are two points I would like to draw from this anecdote. First, it is an illustration of how traumatic episodes create unconscious impressions and memories which can act as triggers for future behaviour (in this case, my aversion for the food). The negative effects produced by these experiences can create internal imbalance and conflict. These conflicting forces, in my opinion, can be a major factor causing disease.

Secondly, traumatic episodes of this type are frequent occurrences on the road to maturity. Some of these experiences can cause deep scars and if these are not neutralized healing cannot fully take place. I feel that the stress produced from this episode and other similar episodes in my life contributed to my asthma. The causes of asthma will be different in different people. Traumas of life can add up and trigger the inherent potential for asthma to manifest. Whatever the causes, the emotional connection must be dealt with if there is to be any lasting cure.

Kindergarten and early school years

During these years I was afflicted with severe bronchitis, and was beginning to suffer from asthma, which resulted in my undergoing frequent medical investigations. Both my adenoids and tonsils were removed, a less common procedure these days.

I went through a series of investigations to determine the substance to which I was allergic, as it was believed that an allergy was the main cause of my illness. Approximately 200 scratches on each forearm were dabbed with allergens. These scratches produced weals (raised red patches) and it was concluded that the largest weal was the allergen causing my sickness. I was injected twice a week with increasing doses of this allergen in an effort to produce immunity in my weakened body.

This painful process went on for six months and was repeated two years later. It failed to have any lasting effect on my bronchitis or asthma. Modern scientific research also

4

holds that the use of these injections is not of any lasting benefit. The science of psychoneuro-immunology agrees with the yogic view that the mind is a more important cause of allergic diseases.

School life

One painful memory stands out from my primary school years. I was progressing rather slowly in school, and one day at the age of ten I heard my parents and teacher discussing my immaturity. I felt hurt and this compounded a negative attitude towards myself. This attitude hampered progress in my healing. It is my belief that positive encouragement is essential for healing.

During this period I was taking many drugs: anti-cough, anti-cholinergics, anti-histamines and nasal decongestants. These drugs seemed to suppress the illness at times but did not remove it; I was still subject to numerous asthma attacks. The slightest exertion would bring on asthma again and again. Eventually I became round-shouldered and developed a slump because of my weak condition.

Beginning of cure

The turning point in my battle with asthma came at the age of eighteen. During that year I entered medical school and at the same time discovered yoga therapy. Yoga seemed the natural direction for me; the people it attracted were happy, friendly and giving. Each yoga teacher I met had something new to offer me, perhaps a humble attitude to life, or just a friendly smile.

I began with some simple asanas (yoga poses). My cure was far from an overnight one. In fact, for a while, my asthma intensified. This intensification was in part due to old tensions which were surfacing and coming to my awareness. Often during a session of yoga, or shortly afterwards, when my mind was in a tranquil state, an old memory would leap into my consciousness with all of its accompanying emotional content.

5

Another obstacle to my progress lay in my own expectations. I had not begun yoga with the express purpose of curing my asthma, but as I began to notice some improvement, I found myself trying too hard with the postures. I was creating tensions instead of easing them. It took some months of effort and frustration before I came to the realization that relaxation is the starting point of therapy. I began to perform the asana and pranayama in a relaxed and cheerful manner, paying less attention to 'progress' and 'improvement'.

In fact, progress began to come of its own accord after this realization. The asanas began to reshape and recondition my body and the pranayama strengthened my lungs.

I now realize that my progress would have been faster if I had been performing a program directly aimed at curing asthma rather than just a general one. There remained many ups and downs on the road to health. A lifetime of conditioning and negative thought and behaviour patterns cannot be overcome in a few days or weeks. However, after only a few years of intensive efforts, I find that today I am completely cured.

Parent-child relationships and asthma

I would like to add some observations on the importance of the parent-child relationship. This is, of course, a familiar subject in psychoanalytic literature but it is especially relevant to the asthmatic. Speaking for myself, I can still recall the pain and stress caused by the absence of my parents and their comforting presence due to their work commitments.

The parents' attitudes towards the child are particularly important. If they project their ambitions onto the child, he or she can very easily become neurotic and insecure.

In this context, I can quote the example of a female friend of mine. She was very intelligent and successful in her studies; however, she was pushed by her parents in directions that were not of her own choosing. She was obliged to study subjects of her parents' choice rather than her own. What is more, her parents expected her to be a great success and made this very clear to her. I feel that this contributed greatly to the psycho-physical stresses that she suffered. It is possible that these types of stresses aggravated her asthma.

When I visited the family, her parents were constantly pressuring her; in fact, in a subtle manner they even criticized her asthma attacks as preventing her from doing her studies. They failed to realize that in their attempts to help her they contributed to her stress. This stopped her from relaxing and also reinforced negative beliefs in herself. Luckily, this friend was able to use yoga to develop positive self-esteem and to grow into a healthy, confident person. Her health improved further when she left home and developed an independent life. Today she is a healthy, successful person who has integrated yoga into her lifestyle.

Many of the ways in which the parent-child relationship can create stress are described by Eric Berne, MD in the book *Games People Play*. For example, Berne gives the game 'Corner': "Corner is a family game involving children, where it resembles the double-bind... Here the small child is cornered so that *everything* he does is wrong... e.g., the child is urged to be more helpful around the house, but when he is, the parents find fault with everything he does."

In the last chapter the author states: "For certain fortunate people there is something which transcends all classification of behaviour and that is awareness; something which rises above the programming of the past and that is spontaneity; and something that is more rewarding than games and that is intimacy. But all three of these may be frightening and even perilous to the unprepared."

These 'games' build up continuously. In the asthmatic they are blocks to health and must be acknowledged, managed and, if possible, removed. Through yoga and the cultivation of awareness which comes from yoga, we are able to deal with, and occasionally remove, the sources of sickness and not just the symptoms.

Concluding note

Internal disease is a state of chaos and imbalance which may reflect the state of external relationships. For an asthmatic whose life is disrupted by disease and who must avoid normal childhood activities, relationships can also be affected and disturbed. This in turn can reinforce negative self-image, which either encourages further illness or prevents one dealing effectively with problems. This is the 'vicious circle' of disease.

As I began to come out of this vicious circle, I learned to use disease and its effects on me in a positive way to learn as much as I could about myself and the world. I was convinced that an important root of disease lies in the subtle regions of the body/mind, and it is here that we can begin to effect a cure. We cannot simply suppress the symptoms in the hope that the disease will go away itself. Positive work must be done to strengthen the mind and body.

The body can be thought of as the earth, the mind as the sea and the emotions as the seashore. If there is turbulence in the sea, it beats on the shore and drags it away from the land. A calm sea results in an untroubled seashore. A calm mind produces a feeling of tranquillity and is itself a healing factor. The emotional person who is worried and anxious may be destroying his body because of an overactive mind. Yoga can calm the mind and heal the body.

2

Some Basics About Asthma

The purpose of this information is to bring the reader to an awareness of the symptoms and condition of asthma. Those who have experienced asthma will, of course, be familiar with these facts, but it is hoped that they will benefit from a logical and ordered presentation of the subject and will be in a position to deal with an attack in a systematic way. Doctors, teachers and other readers will be in a better position to give assistance to those suffering from asthma, who may have an attack in their own vicinity.

The basic cause of an asthma attack is the contraction of the breathing tubes. This is accompanied by overproduction of mucus, further blocking the airway. The attack manifests itself as an excruciating breathlessness, especially during exhalation, producing a wheezing sound.

Basic facts

• Asthma originates most commonly in infancy and less so in middle life.

• It occurs with equal frequency in both sexes during youth. However, males are more susceptible in later life than females.

• There are hereditary factors causing asthma but these do not render a cure impossible.

• Nervousness is intimately linked with the disease. Worry, smoking and pollution are major contributing causes.

- Complications which can result from asthma include bronchitis and, in some cases, emphysema.
- Asthma itself is not fatal. The extreme case, status asthmaticus, results in serious illness but even this condition is reversible.

Asthma can be classified according to the predominant elements of the body – air, fire and water:

1. Air (*vata*) produces a dry asthma with coughing and wheezing but little mucus.
2. Fire (*pitta*) causes inflammation and produces asthma with bronchitis.
3. Water (*kapha*) is the most common form of asthma – a wet type with thick, heavy mucus accompanied by wheezing and coughing.

Asthma with a predominance of the water element often occurs in the cold months of the year when the body builds up excessive amounts of mucus and cannot burn it off. That is, the body does not generate enough internal metabolic heat to handle the cold climate, and as a result mucus builds up and is not expelled from the body. This is combined with spasms of the bronchioles and bronchi (tubes of the lungs), preventing sufficient air getting out. Breathlessness, wheezing, gasping and coughing result.

This condition is aggravated by anything which produces mucus, such as cold, and excessively starchy foods (rice, sweets, milk products, etc.) Ultimately this disease has its roots in the subtle body, i.e. the mind, as well as in the genetics of the body.

The attack

The onset of an asthma attack is usually sudden, but often there are clear warning signs: an allergic attack in a dusty room, a feeling of depression, lethargy, sleepiness, indigestion, a copious flow of mucus in the nose, or an increase in the quantity of urine, perhaps brought on by a stressful situation. During the attack the smooth involuntary muscles of the bronchial tubes constrict and the amount of air going in and out decreases. To try and normalize breathing, the person with asthma consciously starts to use his accessory breathing muscles. He or she tightens the muscles at the base of the neck (including the trapezius) and in trying to force air out, uses all his chest muscles. This creates fatigue, which increases anxiety and weakness. The asthmatic gives the appearance of heaving at every breath.

After some hours, or perhaps even days, the constricted bronchial tubes relax, allowing the sufferer to cough up mucus secretions and sink into an exhausted sleep. Should the asthmatic also suffer from a cold or other respiratory ailments, the attack is even more severe, with delayed recovery and the possibility of bronchitis or pneumonia to follow. Bronchitis is one of the most common complications from asthma.

During asthma the mucus membranes become inflamed and breathing in an attack becomes most difficult. A feeling of suffocation ensues. The sufferer coughs often, usually without success, in an effort to clear the air passage of mucus. In an attempt to get some air into the lungs, the asthmatic must sit up and bend forward. The effect of this can be to create a permanent forward hunch.

Between attacks

The person with asthma has four major problems that confront him between attacks. Each of these predisposes him to another attack. They are:

1. *Debility*: Physical and emotional weakness ensuing from the strain of an asthma attack renders the sufferer vulnerable to another attack. A vicious circle is then easily established.
2. *Inactivity*: Physical debility disrupts work and other activities. This withdrawal from normal activity can bring on depression and thoughts of another attack.
3. *Fear of future attacks*: The vivid memory of the previous attack combines with the sufferer's weakness and inactivity to bring on fears of yet another attack.

11

4. *Postural defects*: The positions adopted by the body during an attack to maintain the flow of air are sometimes retained between attacks and can lead to postural defects. These are magnified by the asthmatic's general physical weakness.

Our purpose is to show how yoga can short-circuit these problems and help prevent further attacks of asthma.

3

The Respiratory System

A knowledge of the structure and function of the respiratory system will enable the reader to visualize exactly what happens during an attack. The unknown is usually much more frightening than the familiar. Increased awareness on the part of the sufferer will allow energy to be directed with greater will and purpose. If a person who has a disorder of any part of his body centres his attention on it with sufficient concentration and combines this with other intervention, in time it will improve its state of health and function.

The organs of respiration

As air is inhaled it passes through the nostrils or the mouth, the larynx and the trachea (or windpipe). Around the middle of the chest the trachea divides into two tubes, called the bronchi. Each bronchus passes to a lung and measures four inches in length. The bronchi divide into small branches, the bronchioles, inside the lungs. These bronchioles transmit air to and from the minute air sacs (alveoli) of the lungs.

The lungs, lying on either side of the chest, are spongy and porous with very elastic tissue. They contain innumerable air cells; if placed in water the lungs would float.

The bronchioles contain circular muscle fibres in their walls and will constrict when these muscle fibres contract. These fibres are activated either locally (e.g. by irritation of the bronchial passages, infection, allergy, etc.) or via the autonomic nervous system, stimulated by tension and other stresses. The constriction of the bronchioles is considered to be a major part of the asthma attack. Within the walls of the tubes of the lungs are various receptors for allergic response to dust, pollen and so on. These play a major role in asthma.

Another obstruction to breathing is blockage by mucus. The walls of the lungs contain two types of glands: mucus secreting and serous secreting. The serous glands secrete a watery fluid but are rarely used in the lungs and are now thought to be the resting stage of the mucus glands. In the healthy lung, the mucus glands are constantly producing a secretion which prevents foreign particles, such as dust and germs, from entering the lung proper. The mucus is moved upwards and out of the lungs by the continuous, rhythmical beating of tiny, hair-like projections from the walls of the tubes. The cough reflex aids this process.

When the disease process sets in, the serous or resting phase of these glands is called into action and the number of mucus glands increases. The mucus becomes copious and stickier so that the tubes block and breathing becomes even more difficult.

Inhalation and exhalation are brought about by the alternate expansion and contraction of the thorax or chest. Three sets of muscles operate during inhalation: the intercostal muscles, (the muscles acting on the ribs), the diaphragm (a large dome-shaped sheet of muscle separating the chest from the abdomen) and the accessory muscles. Contraction of these muscles causes the chest cavity to become deeper, longer and broader, and as a result air is sucked in. The relaxation of these muscles and the elastic recoil of the lungs forces the air out.

Thus, while inhalation is an active process, exhalation is normally a passive process. When there is some obstruction to exhalation the expiratory process must become active. The wall of the abdomen contracts actively, forcing the

14

diaphragm higher and pulling the ribs closer together than usual, forcing out additional air. The muscle groups used in this way tire quickly. An asthmatic tires quickly when forced to expend energy on exhalation. Mucus blockage builds up. Th cough reflex tries to push the mucus out of the system, but due to fatigue, one is less able to expel all of the blockage.

As the expiratory muscles weaken, the sufferer is not able to expel all the air from the lungs and over time the lungs may become distended. The result is increasing breathlessness, poor lung function and anxiety or depression.

The central nervous system

The central nervous system, which controls the body, is located in the brain and spinal column. The peripheral nervous system carries messages to and from voluntary muscles and sensory receptors. The autonomic nervous system regulates and controls involuntary movements of the body, such as heartbeat, normal breathing, intestinal movement and the bronchial tube muscles.

The autonomic nervous system is comprised of the sympathetic and parasympathetic parts. The sympathetic system acts to speed up vital processes while the parasympathetic slows them down. These two systems function automatically and in a healthy person are well coordinated.

The weakness of the breathing mechanism in an asthmatic causes the autonomic nervous system to become unbalanced. Because of ongoing stress in the parasympathetic nervous system it is fatigued and the sympathetic nervous system becomes excessive, rendering the body incapable of coping with stress. Stress, in turn, causes more weakness in the nervous system.

Muscle

Muscle is the basic unit of movement in the body. It is controlled by the nervous system and fed by the blood. There are two types of muscle: skeletal, which is voluntary, and smooth muscles, which ordinarily is involuntary. It is worth noting, however, that through advanced yoga techniques one may influence smooth muscle also.

During an attack the smooth muscle inside the bronchial tubes contracts, permitting less air to pass. Skeletal muscle in the chest wall is also contracted because of panic arising at the onset of the attack.

Blood vessels

Oxygen in the air that is inhaled passes through the thin walls of the air sacs and enters the blood. The blood vessels carry the oxygen throughout the body to nourish it. The first action of a new-born infant is to draw in life-giving breath. Faulty respiration causes insufficient absorption of oxygen into the blood, and also results in the accumulation of waste matter such as carbon dioxide. A city dweller, for example, normally has shallow respiration using only the upper part of the lungs. This, however, can be easily corrected.

Yogic breathing exercises the respiratory muscles and the lungs and opens many of the air sacs which are normally closed. This produces a greater supply of oxygen to the blood. The result is better health and decreased tension and strain.

Lymph vessels

Lymph vessels collect waste material that is not picked up by the blood vessels. Lymphatics, nerves, arteries and veins all run together and are seen as four or five tubes lying side by side. The balanced action of these is essential.

The flow of lymph requires muscle action, such as hard physical exercise. In a city this type of work is not available. Thus, yoga exercises (asanas) take its place.

4

Combating the Effects

We have already mentioned some of the problems that people face after experiencing an attack of asthma. Now we will discuss some ways by which these problems can be overcome.

Posture

Poor posture is a problem with many asthmatics. In some cases, physical weakness causes one to slump over in a permanent round-shouldered position. This puts many other physical structures out of alignment. Poor posture is caused by, and causes, pranic disruption. Energy does not flow smoothly or evenly. Before good health can be restored, these basic deformities need to be addressed and function restored so that prana can begin to flow. Fortunately, the poor posture found in asthma is often easily corrected by yoga. The asanas correct defects while contributing directly to overall health. Pranayama increases prana in the tissues.

The spinal cord carries vital information along its millions of nerve pathways. It is dependent on a supple spine for good nutrition and the flexibility to allow the nerves emerging from it to have a clear and free access to facilitate conduction. In the hunched position the flow of prana along the spine is restricted so that information is often not carried accurately.

People with asthma need to increase their effort to improve the health of their spines. However, they may not

17

feel they have the energy to do this. This may be because breathing takes precedence. In fact, this hunching creates another vicious circle: The chest muscles are pushed over in such a way that the breathing mechanisms lose their efficiency. In addition, the spinal nerves are pinched and constricted. The information going to the brain is that there is a disease in progress: nerves are pinched, the lungs sick, the body weak. Information required for normal function is distorted.

If poor posture is allowed to continue for some time the position becomes harder to remedy. With the onset of old age, the bones in the spine will ossify and correction will be almost impossible. For the healing process to begin, one must realize several things:

• By allowing this process to continue we are doing ourselves harm.

• We need to learn which areas of the body require the most attention. These are areas where awareness should be placed. The simple act of bringing awareness to the parts which need attention (lungs, ribcage, spinal cord, vertebrae and nervous system) will be a positive step. It is worth reiterating that directing positive thoughts to an area will send healing energies to that area.

• Most important, we must give ourselves the positive impetus to begin the healing process. This is the first step out of the vicious circle of disease and we must do this for ourselves.

Suggestions for correcting posture

First of all, chairs can be a hindrance to good posture. Very few chairs are designed to take into consideration the varying needs of those who sit in them. Some attempt can be made to cultivate a comfortable kneeling or cross-legged sitting position on the floor. With time you will be able to sit for longer periods in the position and may find it a preferred way of resting. The important point is to create more options and skills for ourselves. Sitting on the floor has the extra

18

advantage that you can perform asanas at any time, just by moving a leg here or there. For example, when reading, you can move into the crocodile pose (makarasana) if sitting cross-legged is too tiring.

If you do sit in a chair remember to use a good posture. Slouching in chairs is a habit most of us acquired from years of classroom sitting. If you notice that you are slouching, or if the back becomes tired, stretch backwards over the backrest of the chair. A good sigh will release the tension. This can be done gently in order to 'click' the vertebrae. The spinal vertebrae will realign themselves by this movement, freeing up the spinal nerves and making the spine more supple. A series of clicks in the spine is usually accompanied by a deep relaxation of the back, indicating that the spine is well on its way to recovery.

A simple and useful exercise for the spine is as follows: standing with both feet firmly planted on the ground, bring the arms up to shoulder height. Keep the hips firm and motionless and swing the arms around the body. Let this action take the top half of the body, from the waist up, around to its fullest extent. This is kati chakrasana. You can swing the body around once or twice.

Nasal factors in asthma

The nasal passages are part of the same respiratory system as the lungs and are equally subject to the conditions of imbalance present in asthma. In particular, nasal congestion is a common occurrence in asthma.

Many people with asthma breathe through their mouths. In this way they do not allow the air to be warmed by the copious blood supply of the nose, nor to be cleaned of dust and foreign particles by the hairs in the nostrils.

Nose drops, commonly used to relieve nasal congestion, are a poor solution; they only add more toxins to the body and make it work even harder to clean itself. The medical profession itself recommends that these drops be used as little as possible. They can do more harm than good.

19

Instead of drugs, a yoga cleansing technique such as neti should be used. Backward bending asanas help to unclog the blocked nasal compartment. Followed by yoga breathing techniques they can, if practised for some time, bring permanent relief.

Good posture will also help nasal problems. Because the nasal and respiratory passages are in one straight line, hunching of the shoulders hinders the free flow of air from the nose. The air is forced to travel through a bent and constricted passage. The asthmatic should therefore try to keep his head and back straight at all times and breathe through the nose.

The use of drugs

Cure of asthma means, of course, freedom from drugs also. It is our experience that drugs are more often an antidote to fear and anxiety than to any specific disease. The asthmatic reaches for drugs, such as a spray, long before it is necessary. An essential part of the healing process is the breaking of this dependence. It is much better to watch and wait at the onset of an attack, hard as this may be at first. This willpower and positive attitude is the first and most important step on the road to recovery.

5

Probable Causes of Asthma

The cause of asthma is a combination of many factors, including an immunological reaction and overstimulation of the parasympathetic nerve fibres to the lungs, which constricts the bronchial tubes.

The parasympathetic nerves originate in an area of the brain called the hypothalamus, which is directly under the control of higher emotional centres. Hence, emotional tension 'plays on' the hypothalamus which then sends stimuli down the parasympathetic nerve fibre, which can in turn trigger an asthma attack. The cure? Stop the deep mental and emotional reactions and you will stop the asthma. However, this is not easy to do.

The most common illnesses today are psychosomatic diseases. Deep rooted, subtle mental complexes cause disturbances in the emotions and the body. They can cause great bodily changes and muscular tension. Emotional stresses are the surface reflection of deeper processes. They remain with us for some time, until we can deal with them. Few people can get angry or worried and then immediately put aside the experience and regain their equanimity. The yogi, however, can do this. Every thought and emotion we have, in some way affects the body. The best insurance for good health is a calm and quiet mind. For asthmatics, the need for peace of mind, strength and the ability to relax are most important.

21

For example, the feeling which many people have of being tired or worn out all the time is often caused by mental disturbance and emotional factors. There may be a physical reason, such as anaemia; more often, however, factors of which the person is not even aware are important. These can often be revealed to us through the processes of yoga and meditation.

Drugs alone cannot cure asthma; they can only treat the symptoms. Only treatment of the cause can produce a cure. When you have cured asthma with yoga you will no longer need drugs. Western science advances four possible causes of asthma, which are listed below in order of importance:
1. Stress, worry, anxiety and psychosomatic problems
2. Allergy and other irritants
3. Genetic or hereditary characteristics
4. Unknown causes

We shall now discuss each of these causes in terms of both yoga and science.

Stress

The values of today's society produce disharmony and stress, so that many people resort to escape mechanisms to temporarily relieve the distress caused by the turmoil in their lives. They indulge in pastimes and distractions such as television and movies, and habits such as smoking, drinking and overeating to avoid facing themselves and their daily life.

Disease is caused by an unnatural lifestyle. This fact is demonstrated by people like the Hunzas whose natural lifestyle has produced an average lifespan of 100 years. It is possible to lead a relatively natural life even while we go about our work in the city. Factors which will contribute to this are peace of mind, good diet, hard work and plenty of exercise, sun and fresh air. Through initiating a natural lifestyle combined with yoga, the asthmatic can overcome many of the subconscious worries and anxieties which block good health. To do this, he faces a hard but rewarding road.

The mind has many subtle mechanisms which are difficult to detect.

One habit which should be cultivated is that of objectivity or 'mindfulness'. For example, it may happen that an asthmatic is exposed to a painful or difficult situation. If he reacts by thinking, "Oh no! Now I'll get an asthma attack..." then of course he will get an attack. But when he learns habits of calmness and equanimity from yoga practice he will be able to observe the situation, and his own reactions to it, without becoming involved in this build-up of anxiety. He will also be able to discriminate when a real attack is occurring and deal with it better.

We know from experience that this anticipation is a major factor in an attack. We can train our own nervous and immune systems to react to imagined threats.

Allergy and irritants

An allergy is an unusual bodily chemical response to an ordinary stimulus which is harmless in similar amounts for most people. The allergic reaction results from the release of histamines and other chemicals in the body tissue, affecting one or more of the internal organs. In the nose, allergy manifests as hay fever, in the lungs as asthma. Both of these diseases, as well as other allergies such as hives and eczema, are frequently emotional in origin. They are said to be triggered by irritants such as dust, smog and sudden cold, but even in these cases the emotional element is found to be significant.

Hereditary factor

The extent of hereditary influence on asthma is not yet known. Heredity undoubtedly plays a large part in everyone's life. Still, we can either manage or transcend it. All that is needed is conscious awareness and the will to change. It is possible to overcome our problems and redirect the direction which life seems to have set for us. Health can be regained, especially for those with asthma.

Asthma and relaxation

The episode which follows involved a doctor on duty for the night shift at an inner city hospital. He had been particularly busy one night with some emergency procedures. When these were dealt with, most of the staff retired. A few minutes later a patient came to the emergency section suffering from status asthmaticus, the most severe and crippling stage of asthma. The doctor was called for this case and was alone at the time. In the course of the routine preliminary investigation, he placed one hand on the chest of the patient who by now had literally turned blue. Fatigue and strain caused him to fall asleep with his hand still on the patient's chest. After dozing for a few minutes he awoke to find the patient breathing more easily and spontaneously. However, because he had fallen asleep, the doctor panicked and the patient resumed his wheezing and laboured breathing.

Inspired, the doctor resumed his state of relaxation, calming himself and removing all thoughts from his mind. He tried to communicate some of his calmness through his hand to the patient's chest. The patient immediately began to release some of his own tension and to breathe more slowly and steadily. His colour faded from deep blue to pink. His recovery was so rapid that a simpler treatment than that required for status asthmaticus was initiated.

The story of this doctor indicates that the principles of yoga come closer to the truth than the approach of drug therapy. Relaxation is the key to curing asthma.

Yoga and medicine compared

Modern medicine has a wide spectrum of drugs available for the suppression of the symptoms and effects of asthma, but it has no method for effectively curing and preventing it. This can only be done through natural harmonious living combined with relaxation, exercise and a positive attitude to life combined with yoga and meditation.

Of course, drugs are required to relieve suffering and to stop the misery of a severe attack. However, they must be used with the correct attitude and the understanding that they should be used only if necessary. Drugs can provide excellent relief from the breathlessness and anxiety of asthma, but they have drawbacks.

From experience, we have found that relaxation techniques such as yoga nidra and cleansing techniques such as kunjal kriya are very effective in managing asthma, relaxing the bronchial tubes and allowing the clearing of mucus. Although the effects of these techniques are not as pronounced and dramatic as drugs initially, their long-term effect is much more lasting. They enable the person with asthma to relax in the confidence that he will be able to handle an attack should one arise. The patient can adjust his dosages of medication as per the lung function, and increase yoga practice to ultimately free himself from suffering.

6

Medical Treatment

Most people with asthma are involved in one or more medical treatments or are using alternative medicine to ease the symptoms in the hope of a cure. The use of both medical drug regimens and natural therapies is recommended. Both can play an integral part in the treatment of asthma. It is also important to understand how these treatments operate so that the inclusion of yoga into your medical treatment regimen can be made as smoothly and safely as possible. In this regard you should take the advice both of a fully qualified yoga therapist and of your own medical practitioner.

The best results come when you continue both your medication and yoga side by side. Use drugs or therapies until you feel sure that you have learned yoga properly and are practising regularly. At that stage you can begin to modify your drug therapy under the guidance of qualified people, consistently monitoring your progress. There are methods to measure the degree of improvement of your asthma as you progress with yoga. There may be times when improvement takes longer than you might like. It is possible that there may be times when it is even advisable to increase your medication.

The usual medical treatments fall into four categories: broncho-dilators, decongestants, anti-inflammatory agents, and locally active substances.

Medical treatment of asthma is changing rapidly and you are advised to find the correct treatment that suits your individual needs.

It is not recommended for the person with asthma to reduce or discontinue the use of drugs immediately on commencing yoga. This is especially important if the person has been using them over a long period. Many people coming to yoga want to stop their medication, believing that it is bad for them. However, initially it is the reverse. The proper use of medication will allow the person to have healthier lungs, which can practise yoga better. As the practice of yoga therapy becomes established and confidence, experience and skill increase, then it becomes easier to reduce the quantity of drugs being taken. You will need to resort to drugs less and less.

7

Diet and Fasting

Diet is a very important factor in the treatment of asthma. It is necessary to eliminate heavy mucus-forming foods which clog the system and prevent it from functioning smoothly. In the strong constitution of a healthy person, many foods can be eaten that are not possible for someone suffering from disease. Exercise is an important part of maintaining digestion as it helps the digestive tract to move wastes through the system and keeps the body balanced. The person with asthma must remember that he is starting off with imbalances in various bodily systems. He must first regain balance and then strengthen and fortify his system so that balance is maintained.

Initially it may be best to stick to one diet as the basis for your lifestyle. Changes can be made as you feel strength returning. This stable base will allow you to understand more about diet and how it affects you as, with regularity, the effects of each dietary change become more obvious. For example, if you reintroduce rice into your diet, you will be able to see if there is a change in mucus production, breathing and so on. At the same time you can indulge yourself sometimes, guilt free, in a favourite but forbidden delicacy, because the occasional indiscretion does no harm when we have established a regular, healthy staple diet. Our habits will determine whether we will be healthy or plagued with asthma.

28

The best diet for someone suffering from asthma consists of fresh vegetarian food: boiled, steamed or raw vegetables (not fried); fruit; honey; home-made wholemeal bread and other forms of wheat such as chappati, wheatgerm, etc.; barley and other light grains; dal (pulse) such as split peas, mung beans, etc. Legumes like fresh peas, beans, nuts and so on can be eaten when strength returns. Occasionally, other forms of protein may be required to improve strength.

Avoid: heavy wind-producing foods like cabbage, red pumpkin and lentils; starchy foods such as rice and bread from the bakery (particularly white or sandwich bread); dead, processed, artificially coloured and flavoured foods; white sugar; cakes and pastries; processed milk products such as cheese, butter and yoghurt; fried or heavy food. This is especially true for the winter months when mucus production in the body is predominant. Boiled milk and ghee can be used in small amounts.

These suggestions are given only as a guide. It is important not to become too fanatical regarding diet. It is not what one eats occasionally but what and how much is eaten every day that is important. As in everything else, a relaxed, moderate attitude is the best protection against disease.

Overeating

Overeating is a universal malady which people with asthma must be very careful to avoid. Aside from other effects, overeating distends the stomach and limits the downward movement of the abdomen, thus preventing the lungs from expanding fully. The air sacs in the lower part of the lungs (which is the part most used in normal breathing) are constricted and squashed together by the distended stomach. The person with asthma already has some of this space clogged by mucus. Therefore, after overeating, normal breathing becomes a strain on his system. There is also a reflex action of the vagus nerve, which is connected to both the stomach and the lungs. Stress in one part of the system is often reflected as stress in the other.

Overeating is often caused by tension and frustration. Certain needs apparently cannot be fulfilled so the mind tries to fulfil itself by grasping at food. Of course, no fulfilment results from this; the only result is more tension from the stress placed on the stomach. A great deal of willpower is needed to break the overeating habit, but the effort is well worth it. A light, balanced diet is essential for the person suffering from asthma who wishes to regain and maintain good health.

Aids to digestion

These suggestions, if carried out regularly, will aid digestion and conserve the body's energy. They can easily be added to one's daily routine with great benefits.
1. Only eat when hungry.
2. Never overeat.
3. Take small amounts of water during meals. It is important to keep the digestive juices sufficiently concentrated during meals so that digestion may proceed easily.
4. Before and after meals wash the hands, face and mouth.
5. After the meal sit in vajrasana for ten to fifteen minutes. This pose is very helpful for digestion and it relaxes the body.
6. A slow, relaxed walk in the fresh air after a meal is a good way to keep the system ticking over.

Constipation

Constipation, a condition of clogged bowels due to over-dry faeces, can be a contributing factor in asthma. It may result from a sedentary lifestyle, tension, inadequate water consumption, or a faulty diet. The same mechanisms operating in asthma also operate in constipation.

When the bowels are functioning properly, the body is able to remove toxins quickly from the system and bodily processes are maintained at a peak. Constipation is both a symptom of a weak system and another stress on the overburdened system of the asthmatic which contributes to

30

ongoing poor health. It can be reduced by following these suggestions:

1. On rising from bed drink two glasses of warm water with a little lemon juice.
2. Drink plenty of water during the day. Many people are constantly dehydrated from not drinking enough water. Dark, sparse urine is a sign of dehydration. At least one cup of water should be taken between each meal and more as weather conditions warrant.
3. Eat plenty of fresh fruits, particularly papaya and prunes.
4. Vegetables will add the necessary bulk to keep the peristalsis going. Excessive white bread or thick, sticky foods have the opposite effects.
5. Asanas help to remove constipation and tone the entire digestive system.
6. Use meditative practices and gentle pranayama to reduce neuromuscular tension.

Fasting

Fasting is beneficial and in fact necessary for the asthmatic. As a rule, people tend to eat too much and rest too little, a pattern which can only produce tension. Many people eat in excess. Two meals a day are sufficient. In addition, most asthmatics have taken drugs for many years. Toxins may build up in their systems and cause further imbalance. Fasting is a good way to deal with these problems. By fasting we do not mean 'forty days and forty nights' without food, but a gradual, gentle program designed to restore purity to the body. Asthmatics will find that the fast, especially during an acute attack, will produce dramatic effects and remove a great deal of mucus from the lungs, allowing them to breathe freely and effortlessly. For removing mucus from the lungs, the combination of fasting with asana practice is ideal.

Specific benefits from fasting include losing weight and waste in the form of toxins, relaxed breathing, extra energy and decreased mental pressure and tension. Experience will demonstrate the benefits of fasting.

Persons who have taken many drugs or who are debilitated and weak should take particular care while fasting. Fasting is a good method only if used correctly; it can produce harmful effects otherwise. If there are many toxins in the system, a sudden fast can cause the release of too many toxins for the body to handle, causing great discomfort, even disease. This can happen if the asthmatic fasts for too long or if, while fasting, does too many asanas too quickly. The process should be slow and steady. Fasting regularly for a short period has the same effect as a long fast; even missing one meal now and then makes the body healthier and stronger. One main meal a day is a good idea and in itself can improve health.

While fasting, great care should be taken with the practice of asanas. Although they are usually easier to perform during a fast, this does not mean that they should be done more rapidly or for a longer period of time than usual. In fact, they should be done more slowly and with shorter total duration (particularly inverted asanas) to avoid releasing too many toxins at once.

Fasting is best in warm weather when less body heat is required. One day a week is sufficient; later, if desired, the duration of the fast may be increased. The day of fasting should be a day of peace and quiet, with as little mental or physical activity as possible. This will allow more energy to be directed to the parts of the body needing repair.

Immediate fasting is recommended in the case of an acute attack. An attack indicates that the body is in a state of debility and tension, and that possibly excessive toxins have built up. Not only will fasting gradually alleviate the symptoms, it will also help to release tensions stored in the nervous system. The effects of fasting are not as immediate as those of drugs, but the overall results are more beneficial. Again we caution, however, that the fast should not be continued for too long. If weakness and the need for nutrients are felt, then one should eat a small meal.

Fasting for beginners

Those who are new to the practice should fast from lunchtime to lunchtime. This '24 hour fast' places the sleeping period in the middle of the fast and allows the effects of the fast to go on without too many hunger pains. The evening meal should be replaced by water, light tea or fruit juice. By lunch the following day the body will be rejuvenated by its 24 hour fast and will be ready for its next meal.

With all fasts it is best to observe the following procedures:

• The final meal before the fast should be light so that the stomach begins to adjust to a feeling of emptiness.
• During the fast one should drink more water than usual but not to excess. This will wash the system of toxins and flood the kidneys, cleaning and revitalizing them.
• The meal after the fast should be light so that the system may gradually adjust.
• Asthmatics should not attempt fasts of longer than two days until their strength returns. We will give a few recommendations for longer fasts, but urge you to seek expert and personal guidance if you are contemplating a fast of more than three days.

A longer fast should only be contemplated in warm weather, when one has a period of time to totally rest. During the first three days, when the hunger pangs are the worst, fruit or juices (vegetable or fruit) can be taken occasionally. If it is possible a complete water fast is best. Laghoo shankhaprakshalana and enemas may be used to keep the colon clean and maintain constant removal of toxins.

On breaking a long fast, one should drink orange or lemon juice, eat a light, simple diet for a few days, and gradually readjust to a solid diet. A good tonic when the fast is over consists of equal quantities of lemon juice, olive oil and honey. One glass a day is recommended.

The integrated diet

By combining the suggestions on diet and fasting given in this section into your daily routine, you will gain an increased amount of energy and vitality. The recommended diet is both nutritious and adequate to meet the daily needs of most people and at the same time economizes on digestive energy, sending more for healing the devitalized lungs and nervous system. The results of the change in diet may not be apparent initially, but a few months will prove its efficacy as a matter of personal experience. Food is a vital part of our lives and we must learn to use it, or not use it, scientifically and wisely.

8

Yogic Treatment

Most people in the throes of an acute illness will do anything to find relief, usually in the form of drugs and other remedies designed to suppress symptoms. From the yogic and natural health point of view, this can be a mistake. The disease is an attempt by nature to rebalance and heal the body, ridding it of accumulated toxins, chemicals and waste products that have been stored and are clogging vital capillary, lymphatic, nervous and organic channels. These impurities disturb physiological function, converting it to the pathological, and distorting pranic energy fields. The mind is affected in a reciprocal interchange with distorted body energies creating pain, tension and suffering. Disease is nature's mechanism to right the capsizing human vessel and to restore normal function. The process must be aided, not suppressed, so that it takes place in the shortest possible time with maximum benefit and minimum suffering. Yoga achieves this lofty aim.

In this book we are presenting those methods which are best suited to the treatment, based on our direct experience. All the practices listed below are described in the 'Practice' sections of this book. The treatment of asthma through yoga is an involved process and the programs given here should act as guidelines only. The management of asthma should not be attempted without the direct guidance of an experienced yoga teacher.

Topics covered include: cleansing techniques, asana, pranayama, relaxation, yogic attitude and ashram program. Two aspects of cure are considered:
1. Practices to be used during an acute attack.
2. Long-term practices to reduce further attacks.

Only through consistent, steady practice of these exercises is complete recovery brought about. A few minutes of relaxed practice each day is far more preferable to irregular practice of long duration. Bear in mind the fable of the tortoise and the hare. You will find that effort diminishes and relaxation increases as the practices are established on a regular basis.

Cleansing techniques

The hatha yoga cleansing techniques are probably the most important aspect of therapy for asthma. Their salt cleans out the accumulated thick mucus, dissolving it and drawing it out by osmotic force. For people with asthma the salt used in these practices can be slightly increased.

The following techniques should ideally be performed in the morning before asana and meditation practice. Their application during an acute attack is extremely beneficial.

1. *Kunjal kriya* consists of drinking warm, salty water and then regurgitating it by stimulating the back of the throat with the fingers. The effect of kunjal on an acute attack of asthma cannot be underrated. The nervous energy, which is causing many of the symptoms of an attack, can be released with the expulsion of water from the stomach. There is a reflex action from the stomach to the lungs via the vagus nerve, which removes tension from the lungs. If practised regularly, kunjal is beneficial in preventing an attack.

2. *Jala neti* involves washing the nasal passages with warm, salty water. It is of importance to the person with asthma as mouth breathing is a common problem. Neti removes obstructions from the nasal passages and facilitates nasal breathing. Regular practice allows pranayama to be

36

performed more effectively. Once pranayama is practised on a regular basis, the nasal passages will regain even greater health and will remain open longer and longer, so that neti may eventually be discontinued. If the nose is blocked, perform jala neti each day for at least a month to clear the nasal passages. There are three types of neti:

i) *Jala neti* (water neti), using a pot with a spout which fits into the nostril,

ii) *Sutra neti* (catheter neti), done before jala neti, especially when the passages are too blocked to pass water,

iii) *Vyutkrama kapalbhati* (sinus cleansing), passing water in through the nose and out through the mouth.

3. *Vastra dhauti* is done by swallowing a strip of fine muslin about 2½ centimetres wide and up to three metres long. The cloth must be removed from the stomach within twenty minutes. This practice can be followed by kunjal and neti kriyas. Some people find vastra dhauti a great help, others not. You should try it yourself to see if it brings you relief. In many ways, it is more powerful than kunjal. If the strip of cloth is soaked in midstream urine before swallowing, it is said to be even more powerful. During the acute situation it can be used every day for up to two weeks, but after this once a week is sufficient. Of course, this varies from individual to individual.

4. *Shankhaprakshalana* is a very powerful technique for cleaning the whole alimentary canal. It involves drinking a large quantity of salty water, alternated with a series of five asanas. Laghoo shankhaprakshalana is the short form of this technique in which a smaller amount of water is drunk but the same series of asanas is performed. This can be practised during the acute attack and also on a daily basis during the acute situation. By removing the mucus from the intestinal walls, it has a reflex effect on all the mucus glands of the body. The salt absorbed helps to dissolve accumulated mucus in the lungs and other bodily organs and relaxes the nervous system. This

technique is very tiring; after performing it, rest is required. Food restrictions must be followed after full shankhaprakshalana, but not after the short form.

It is important to note that these techniques must not be attempted without expert guidance. If practised daily, the following precautions should be observed:

- They should be done early in the morning when the stomach is empty.
- After performing laghoo shankhaprakshalana and kunjal, one should wait for at least half an hour before eating.

Asana

Asanas give both strength and relaxation to the body. By squeezing the tissue like a sponge and directing the blood flow specifically to certain parts, they help to wash the toxins out of the joints, cavities, tissues, and organs. They act to support the balancing and distribution of prana in the tissues. They also act on much deeper levels, bringing about significant benefits over a long period of time. For the person with asthma, regular practice of asanas will help to reshape the chest, improve posture, strengthen the spinal cord, aid the flow of nervous energy, and rebalance the whole body.

There are many asanas which can be performed with great benefit by the person with asthma; however, we feel that the following are most effective: surya namaskara, marjari-asana, shashankasana, shashank bhujangasana, bhujangasana, pranamasana, sarvangasana, paschimottan-asana, yogamudrasana, dhanurasana, shavasana and ardha matsyendrasana.

Although all of these asanas are beneficial, some will be more suitable than others for each individual. Therefore, it is best to select a few which seem to give you the most benefit and cultivate the practice of these exclusively. For example, one person with asthma found that four asanas (sarvangasana, paschimottanasana, dhanurasana and ardha matsyendrasana) were sufficient.

38

People who have not yet practised asanas may find their bodies too stiff to attempt these asanas immediately. In this case the pawanmuktasana series should be practised for some time to limber up the body.

Pranayama

Pranayama is an excellent means of dealing with tensions. By exercising and strengthening the lungs, rebalancing the autonomic nervous system, and strengthening the entire nervous system, it diminishes the possibility of a future asthma attack. Essentially pranayama is designed to allow us to master the body's energy systems. The practices lead to increased self-confidence and mastery of mind. Through greater control of prana, we gain greater control over ourselves.

Pranayama is best practised regularly after asana. Here are some simple exercises:

1. Inhale slowly, counting the pulse at the inner wrist for six beats or more on inhalation. Exhale for the same number of beats. This can be done for up to twelve beats of the heart for each inhalation and exhalation. After some time the heart and breath will slow down considerably.

2. Nadi shodhana stage 2 (alternate nostril breathing) is very beneficial during the acute attack as well as on a daily basis. See the 'Practices' section.

3. Mild bhastrika (bellows breath) will strengthen the lungs. Combined with kumbhaka (breath retention) it is a powerful means of preventing an attack as it opens all alveoli of the lungs, expels gas and phlegm, increases oxygen in the blood and brings about deep relaxation.

The following practices are a combination of asana and pranayama which have been found to be very useful in the treatment of asthma:

1. Stand erect, with the feet together and arms beside the body. Breathing slowly and deeply, raise both arms in front of the body to shoulder level, then slowly move them outward, sideways and slightly backward. Breathe

39

out while lowering the arms to the sides of the body. Do this five times.

2. Hasta utthanasana.
3. Utthita lolasana.
4. Stand erect, feet together and arms at the side of the body. Inhale deeply, hold the breath, and with the fingers tap all over the chest and sides of the body, gently but firmly, for as long as possible before exhaling. Repeat this a total of five times.
5. Standing as before, inhale, then exhale through the mouth in short bursts with a *ha-ha-ha* sound. Perform five times.
6. Standing erect in the same position as before, inhale deeply, then exhale through the mouth with teeth together, making a hissing sound. Do this five times.
7. Yogic breathing, performed in shavasana, should be done during relaxation periods or in any position when an opportunity arises to breathe consciously.
8. Lying in shavasana, bring the arms over the head onto the floor. (The legs may also be bent and the feet placed on the floor in front of the buttocks.) Take hold of the left elbow with the right hand, and the right elbow with the left hand keeping both arms on the floor. Practise yogic breathing. This posture encourages the fullest, deepest breath, particularly into the clavicular region at the top of the lungs.

When these practices have been perfected, the following pranayamas can be taken up:

1. Advanced stages of nadi shodhana and bhastrika are very beneficial.
2. Kapalbhati (frontal brain cleansing) is a slightly more advanced pranayama technique, which is effective in strengthening the lungs. By stressing exhalation, it reverses the normal emphasis of respiration and completely empties stale air from the lungs. In this respect it is especially good for asthma as the main problem here is difficulty in exhaling.

3. Ujjayi pranayama (the psychic breath) increases the intake of oxygen, calming and revitalizing the nervous system. It rebalances the sympathetic and parasympathetic components, which are unbalanced in asthma, and thereby restores harmony.
4. Bhramari (humming bee breath) pranayama is more a relaxation technique than a pranayama.

Pranayama practices are very powerful and the beginner is cautioned not to perform these techniques too forcibly until the body is sufficiently prepared.

Relaxation

One of the best ways of combating asthma is the method of yoga nidra or psychic sleep, the state of inner awareness combined with complete relaxation. In this scientifically proven method of relaxing tensions the student allows the body to sleep but maintains complete control of the mind, moving the awareness from point to point in a systematic way. A guide is usually required in the beginning, but with practice the person with asthma will be able to use it independently in times of stress. In case of an attack, the mental attitude gained in yoga nidra helps to relax the spasm in the chest and lungs. In the normal situation it can be practised just before retiring to produce a deep sleep. Fewer hours of sleep will be required and you will awake feeling fresh and energetic.

Om chanting is a simple yet powerful practice which is very helpful to the person with asthma. Om can be chanted at different speeds. To chant slowly, breathe in fully and deeply. Form the mouth in the shape of an 'O' and in a relaxed way slowly allow the air to escape through the throat making this sound. When the air is almost exhausted, make the 'mmmmm' sound. The process is natural and relaxed. Chant Om loudly at first; later you may continue to repeat it mentally. It is best to practise in a sitting or meditation posture. Let yourself go during the practice and continue it as long as you wish. Try to become absorbed in the mantra.

The person with asthma will find that along with numerous spiritual benefits, Om chanting is most relaxing and strengthening. The vibrations emanating from this mantra will produce a gentle massaging effect which can later be directed to any part of the body that is desired.

Yogic attitude

Attitude is the prime factor in the cure. The person with asthma needs to make an honest self-appraisal to decide whether he really wants to be cured. He must then set his own health as a central priority in life. This requires commitment, sincerity, self-responsibility and intelligent effort.

Yoga treatment requires a certain amount of time each day. Nothing will be accomplished overnight, and damage can easily result from trying to do too much too quickly. It is therefore recommended that a fixed amount of time be set aside each morning for practising and that this time be regarded as inviolate. This may require going to bed an hour or so earlier each night, but in the long run it will prove beneficial.

Once the program is underway, the sufferer – who, from the yogic point of view, is a self-healer – faces further tests of attitude and will. Old memories and volitions will begin to surface, bringing on tension and emotional suffering. These incidents may be a sign that cure is progressing. It is often good to talk to a therapist about these experiences for confirmation. The sufferer should remember that the most important thing is to remain aware all the times.

What is awareness? At the simplest level it is bare attention, the noting of events without attachment or aversion. One ceases to be 'the sufferer' and becomes 'the observer', noting bodily changes, mental states, and feelings, without identifying with them.

Awareness is a skill, like any other and must be developed. This can be done while sitting quietly, riding in a bus, waiting in a queue, or getting a haircut. Sit or stand comfortably and keep the attention on the rising and falling of the abdomen. Try not to think of the 'rising' or 'falling'; just be aware of the movement of rising and falling. If your attention is distracted by a thought, as soon as you recollect yourself, make a mental note, 'thinking'. If you feel irritation or impatience make a mental note, 'feeling'. If a noise catches your attention, 'hearing' and so on, but always bring the attention gently back to the rising and falling of the abdomen. If you feel frustration, note 'frustration'. If frustration continues, stop the practice for the time being and try again later.

Awareness and a positive attitude towards cure can transform your entire life. You will soon come to view situations as learning experiences rather than annoyances. The overcoming of asthma is a big achievement and should be undertaken with energy and a cheerful optimism.

Asthma program

We conclude this chapter with a brief description of the treatment program for asthma used at the Bihar School of Yoga, Munger, India. Although it is quite possible to begin the healing process while carrying on a householder life, it is our experience that the combination of discipline, energy and serenity in the ashram environment are very conducive to cure. In addition, the asthmatic can be sure of expert guidance which will lead him step by step on the road back to health.

The ashram program for asthmatics is as follows:
• *Day 1–4*: Cleansing techniques are begun along with a strict diet and gentle asanas. Each morning vastra dhauti is practised, followed by kunjal kriya and neti kriya. Only the pawanmuktasana part 1 and 2 series of asanas and pranayama are used while the patient's condition is weak.
• *Day 5*: Everyone remains silent on this day and shankha-prakshalana is performed. The remainder of the day is used for resting.
• *Following days*: Japa, antar mouna and yoga nidra are introduced. Surya namaskara is begun gently, usually

43

three rounds a day until the patient shows signs of strength. As progress is made, the asana and pranayama practices increase in number and strength. Later the powerful healing technique known as prana vidya may be given.

All these practices are given under personal guidance in the ashram and tailored to suit individual needs. Some people begin the more advanced practices straight away and have amazingly rapid results. Others require months of simple practices and slow painstaking work. The ashram environment is a great aid in yoga therapy for it allows people to come face to face with themselves and see just what is the basic problem, past experience or conditioning which caused their asthma in the first place. Ashram life takes one to the root cause of the problem.

9
Practice Programs

For the acute attack

What is experienced during an acute attack of asthma? We can answer this question generally: usually there is panic and confusion in the mind with many mixed feelings of fear, pain and misery. Each sufferer, however, has his own version of this experience. At the same time each disease has its own specific characteristics, dependent on such factors as the individual's personality, temperament, genetic constitution, environmental upbringing, past karma and so on. If asthma is to be cured, each aspect of it must be carefully and dispassionately examined. What exactly do you experience during an acute attack? What are your thoughts, memories, feelings and states of mind? Observe yourself during an attack; remain aware of all your internal processes.

When you think you are going to have an acute asthma attack, you can do the following:

1. Sitting on a chair, or at the side of your bed, bend over so that your elbows are on your knees. The chin can rest in the palms of the hands or the hands can be placed between the knees. The shoulders, chest and whole body should be relaxed. Relax into this position and try to feel the breath freeing up.

2. Alternatively, you can perform pranamasana (bowing pose) with the hands by the head. Shashankasana is also

45

a valuable relaxation exercise in the early stages of an attack. These positions allow us to relax and breathe more easily.

3. Control the breath in each of these positions by performing 5 counts inhalation, 5 counts internal retention and 5 counts exhalation. Try external retention for 5 counts if it is possible. Continue this for at least 10 minutes.

If the above practices are used as soon as you feel an attack coming on, then you may be able to abort the attack. However, if it continues, salt therapy is probably the best means to unclog the pipes of the lungs, relax the nervous system and remove mental tensions. This is achieved through the practices of laghoo shankhaprakshalana, kunjal, neti and vastra dhauti. Salt is one of the most curative substances for the patient with asthma. It enters the body and draws out the mucus and reduces inflammation, thereby removing discomfort.

If you feel the acute asthmatic attack progressing, perform the following:

1. Laghoo shankhaprakshalana, if there is sufficient warning before an attack builds up (to whatever extent is possible for your physical condition).

2. Kunjal kriya should be practised after completing laghoo shankhaprakshalana. Kunjal on its own is a very effective counter for the acute asthmatic attack.

3. Then do jala neti and kapalbhati.

4. Practise pranayama or Om chanting. Continue for 5–10 minutes and repeat hourly.

5. If you are not a regular coffee drinker, a hot cup of strong, black coffee taken half an hour after laghoo shankhaprakshalana and kunjal kriya will loosen the spasms, warm the chest and bring relief.

We have found that the acute asthmatic attack is very effectively managed with the above techniques. In one case, a young girl aged 18 had been suffering from asthma since the age of 9 years. She had been undergoing cortisone therapy, but even with this powerful drug she found no relief from her asthma, with her usual attack lasting 7 days. Remarkably, after using this method of treatment, she was relieved of acute asthma in only 2 days.

Therapeutic yoga programs

Between attacks, the following therapeutic practice programs have been found to be very useful in the treatment of asthma and for strengthening the body and mind so that attacks become progressively less frequent and less severe. You will find that yoga practices are not difficult. Given the time and necessary effort required you will be richly rewarded by the beneficial changes that they can bring about.

However, yoga practices are powerful in their effects, bringing about subtle yet profound changes in the body and mind. Therefore, they should be chosen appropriately and practised properly, otherwise the desired effect will not be achieved and under some circumstances there may be an adverse effect. A yoga therapy program should be individually prescribed for each person and supervised by a qualified yoga teacher. At the same time the practices themselves should be learned correctly and practised in a relaxed manner.

The yoga programs outlined here are in three stages, with each consecutive stage including more advanced practices. At least 3 months is recommended for each stage, and that can be extended according to individual needs. You should move on to the next stage of the program only after you can do all the practices from the previous stage with ease, without any physical or mental strain, for a period of at least one month. This will ensure the greatest therapeutic benefits. As your familiarity with the practices grows you will be able to adjust the program according to your needs. In stages two and three, practices from the first stage can continue to be incorporated; their value and effect should not be overlooked

These programs address those people who have uncomplicated asthma, that is without any associated disorders,

47

such as high blood pressure or heart disease. If you have any medical problems apart from asthma, you should consult a qualified yoga therapist for proper guidance. However, all the practices in stage one, if practised in the correct way, are safe in nearly all circumstances. Check the contra-indications for all practices where necessary.

Remember that it is not the quantity but the quality of practice that counts. A few minutes of relaxed and deep practice is worth half an hour of hurried effort aimed at getting as much as possible into the shortest possible time. A relaxed, calm attitude of mind is the aim of the practices and this has to be cultivated over a period of time.

Some mornings we may only have 10 minutes to spare, other times we may have half an hour or more. The ideal situation is to have a set time and place for practice; however, this may not be practical for most people. We should at least practise every day even if only for a few minutes. After initial exposure to the practices, you can aim to design a series that fits your own needs as far as time, social commitments, personal preferences and other variables will allow.

Stage 1: Long program
Jala neti: daily
Hasta utthanasana: 6 rounds
Tadasana: 3 rounds
Trikonasana (from variation 3 go gradually into variations 1 and 2): 3 rounds
Utthita lolasana: 5 rounds
Kati chakrasana: 5 rounds
Pawanmuktasana part 1 (practices for legs, arms and neck on alternating days) 6–10 rounds
Pawanmuktasana part 2 – utthanpadasana: 5–10 rounds; chakra padasana: 5–10 rounds; pada sanchalanasana: 5–10 rounds
Marjari-asana: 5–10 rounds
Sphinx: 3 rounds
Shashankasana: static for 10–27 abdominal breaths

48

Meru wakrasana: 5 rounds
Abdominal breathing: 11 rounds
Yogic breathing in shavasana: 27 rounds
Nadi shodhana: techniques 1 and 2, 1:1 – 5 rounds, gradually
    extending count to 10:10
Bhramari: 9 rounds or ujjayi: 5 minutes
Moola bandha: technique 1–10 rounds
Relaxation/yoga nidra

Stage 1: Short program
Tadasana: 5 rounds
Trikonasana or tiryaka tadasana: 3 rounds ˙
Kati chakrasana: 5 rounds
Pawanmuktasana part 1, shoulder rotation: 5 rounds
Marjari-asana: 10 rounds
Shashankasana: 5 rounds
Pranayama, shatkarma and yoga nidra as in long program

Stage 2: Long program
Jala neti: daily; sutra neti: if necessary 1–4 times a month
Kunjal: once a week, and when necessary
Laghoo shankhaprakshalana: twice a week for one month,
    then can be reduced to once a week
Pada hastasana: 3 rounds static
Dwikonasana: 3 rounds
Pawanmuktasana part 3: kashtha takshanasana: 6 rounds
Surya namaskara: 3–5 rounds
Shavasana with abdominal breath until breath returns to
    normal
Pawanmuktasana part 3: nauka sanchalanasana: 5–8 rounds
Shashank bhujangasana: 5 rounds
Sarpasana: 3 rounds
Utthan pristhasana: static, 10 breaths
Pranamasana: 2 rounds for 10 breaths
Shava udarakarshanasana: 1 round each side
Agnisar kriya (start with swana pranayama for 1 month, then
    move on to actual kriya): 3–5 rounds for 10–20 breaths

Kapalbhati: 3–5 rounds for 20 breaths
Nadi shodhana: technique 2, 1:2 (start with comfortable count, gradually extend to 10:20)
Bhramari: 9 rounds or ujjayi: 5 minutes
Moola bandha: technique 2, 10 rounds with breath synchronization
Relaxation/yoga nidra
Ajapa japa, technique 1 (frontal passage, stages 1,2 and 3) – one month of each stage: 10–15 minutes in the evening

Stage 2: Short program
Shashank bhujangasana: 8 rounds
Sarpasana: 5 rounds
Pranamasana: 3 rounds
Shava udarakarshanasana: 1 round
Pranayama, meditation and shatkarmas as in long program of stage 2

Stage 3
Shatkarmas: as in stage 2
Surya namaskara: 3–8 rounds
Shavasana
Kandharasana: 3 rounds
Paschimottanasana: 2 rounds, static
Gomukhasana: 1 round each side
Yogamudrasana: 2 rounds
Dhanurasana: 3 rounds
Shashankasana, static: 10–27 abdominal breaths
Ardha matsyendrasana: 1 round each side (starting with simple variation)
Sarvangasana/vipareeta karani asana: 1 round (depending on the flexibility of the body)
Matsyasana: 2 rounds
Bhastrika: 3–5 rounds for 20 breaths
Nadi shodhana: stage 3, 1:1:1, gradually build up to 1:1:2 – 5 rounds
Tadagi mudra: 3 rounds

Relaxation/yoga nidra
Ajapa japa, technique 2 (spinal passage, stages 1,2 and 3) –
   one month of each stage: 10–20 minutes in the evening

Note: Please read the introductory notes to the 'Practices'
section. These guidelines apply to both asthma and diabetes.

10

Other Treatments

To gain a broader perspective we are outlining here some of the other known treatments for asthma. Although it is our basic assertion that yoga therapy is sufficient for healing, we also feel that it is important to know something about every avenue available. We acknowledge the use of the book *Asthma, Its Cause and Treatment* by Swami Sivananda Saraswati of Rishikesh for much of this material. The topics covered in this chapter include: coffee cure, herbs, massage, sauna, ayurveda, homeopathy, biochemical salt treatment, speleotherapy and auto urine therapy.

Coffee cure

Coffee is the best drink for the person suffering from asthma. However, it cannot be effective if it is used excessively. Its optimal effect will be felt if it is used only when it is necessary. During the acute attack, a cup of strong black coffee is very beneficial, especially half an hour after the practice of kunjal and neti kriyas. The heat from the coffee has a soothing effect on the stomach, throat and lungs. Coffee is also a mild broncho-dilator because of the amount of caffeine it contains. Therefore, coffee relaxes the nerves and muscles of the bronchial passages, further easing and normalizing the constricted respiration of the asthmatic.

Herbs

We mention here two herbal teas of benefit to the person with asthma:

- *Coltsfoot*: Steep a teaspoon of leaves in a cup of boiling water. Let this stand for a few minutes and drink whenever you like. This herb can also be smoked with great benefits.
- *Dandelion root*: Cut up finely, place in boiling water and drink a few cupfuls a day.

For more information, refer to the extensive literature on herbal medicine. This field is vast, and each herb or combination of herbs can bring about surprising results.

Massage

Massage brings relaxation and rejuvenation to each part of the body. It helps remove aches from joints and sore muscles, as well as contributing to the removal of toxins. Certain forms of massage, such as Ayurvedic and Chinese, are therapeutic and can remove excessive heat and damp which contribute to asthma.

Sauna

Sauna affects the body in much the same way as massage. It is a wonderful method of relaxing and clearing out tensions. Saunas have long been in use and are very popular in Western countries.

In the sauna bath, the external heat sends the blood to the skin and opens the pores. Dirt and other impurities close to the surface now have easy access to the surface of the skin. After a few minutes of sauna (before feeling tired or weak) one should immediately take a cold shower. This prevents impurities from going back in and washes them away. The cold also constricts the outer blood vessels, sending blood to the internal organs.

One should go at once from the shower back into the sauna, bringing more impurities to the surface to be washed away by the cold water. The process should be continued for up to three rounds of hot and cold treatment, each

53

lasting about ten minutes. The cold water is especially beneficial to the asthmatics as it stimulates deep breathing. Hot showers can be used as a substitute for sauna. Take a hot shower, making the water as hot as you can stand, for as long as is comfortable. Then quickly turn on the cold water for the same length of time. Repeat as many times as desired. We recommend that every hot shower be terminated by a cold one. After a few days people with asthma will find this a pleasure rather than a duty. When the shower is over, the body feels alive and active. The cold shower strengthens the entire constitution and helps to combat colds and infection.

Ayurveda

Ayurveda has a history almost as long as that of yoga. To master this discipline would require a lifetime. We can only give a brief idea here of the ayurvedic approach to asthma.

Swami Sivananda Saraswati, in his book *Asthma, Its Cause and Treatment*, states: "Asthma is the disease concerning the five vital airs: prana, apana, udana, samana and vyana. Of these, it has a very close relationship with prana and udana. Ayurveda propounds that there are three main elements in the human body: vata, pitta and kapha – air, bile and phlegm. Vata intensifies kapha and puts obstacles in the path of food, water and air. It dries up the ojas (energy) in the heart. The disease is concerned with difficulty in breathing and it affects the lungs also."

According to ayurveda, some of the causes of asthma are pollution, drinking very cold water, excessive sexual intercourse, excessive travel, excessive fasting, excessive use of spices, oil or tobacco, eating meat, heavy foods which are difficult to digest and fatty foods such as milk products, too many sweets, a strong blow to the chest and so on.

The manifestations of the disease are pain in the chest, pain and constipation in the abdomen, lethargy, excessive dirt in the nasal passages, pain in breathing especially during the night.

54

Some of the treatments are listed below. For more details refer to an ayurvedic text.

1. First, keep the person in a well-ventilated room. Reassure him and cheer him up. Using pillows for support, raise the head, chest and arms. During the day give warm food and drinks, nothing cold. Heat to the chest (for example, a sunbath or a hot water bottle) is a good way to discharge phlegm and bring relief. The evening meal should be as light as possible so that sleep is easier.

2. During and after the attack give only light food: barley water, wheat (dahlia), grapes, raisins, apples, honey and other light and sensible foods.

3. In the hot months give a cold bath and in cold months a warm bath. Open air walks in the early morning are advised.

4. Encourage perspiration (e.g. with hot baths, saunas, sunbaths, blankets, hot drinks) as it helps to remove phlegm and wind.

5. A good drink to give consists of equal parts of honey and ginger juice with some turmeric added. This removes phlegm and mucus and warms the body.

Homeopathy

In homeopathic treatment no harsh drugs are used. The three principles underlying the system are:

1. Like cures like.

2. The magic of the minimum dose (a high potency microdose).

3. Treat the patient and not the disease.

Many people report that in the hands of a trained homeopath this treatment can work wonders.

Biochemical salt treatment

This theory, presented by Dr Schuessler, asserts that disease is partially caused by a deficiency in certain mineral salts which are required by the body in small concentrations. One of the first requirements for the cure of asthma, therefore, is the replenishing of the appropriate salts in the body. The main salts used in this treatment are:

- *Kali Phos.*: This is the chief remedy for obstructed breathing. Take frequently in large doses, especially 'when the asthma is caused by diet'.
- *Kali Mur.*: This treats asthma with thick mucus, constipation and sluggish liver.
- *Kali Sulph.*: For bronchial asthma with yellow sputum.

Other salts which can be effective in treating asthma include: Calcarea Phos. Calcarea Fluor. Natrum Mur., Magnesia Phos. and Natrum Sulph. For full details consult the appropriate text.

Speleotherapy

Salt is a very important component in the treatment of asthma as was mentioned in the section on hatha yoga cleansing techniques. Doctors in Russia have reported on the use of salt in the treatment of asthma. It is reported that many of the people treated for bronchial asthma in the Solotvico Allergologic Hospital in the Ukranian Republic check out in perfectly good health. The hospital is situated deep underground, 300 metres below the surface. The presence of highly saturated sodium chloride acrosol in the mine atmosphere favourably affects the bronchial pulmonary system. It cleans it of all foreign toxins and irritating materials which stagnate in the asthmatic's lungs. Salt seems to help dissolve these out with the mucus.

Auto-urine therapy

Though there is as yet no scientific backing for this ancient technique, auto-urine therapy (*amaroli*) is said to be a wonderful adjunct in the treatment of asthma and other diseases. We have found from personal experience that this technique can help and so we leave it up to you to find out whether it is suitable for you.

The use of this therapy is mentioned in the *Damara Tantra*, where it is called *shivambu kalpa vidhi*, the process of changing and revitalizing the body through the drinking of one's own urine. It is also mentioned in the *Hatha Yoga Pradipika* in the technique of amaroli. Some people even believe it is mentioned in the *Bible* (Proverbs 5:15) where it states, "Drink the water of your own cistern." Many great sages have recommended this therapy.

There are many points for the utilization of urine therapy in the treatment of asthma. Some people say that urine contains cortisone metabolites. Cortisone is a drug produced in the body, but given in tablet form in the treatment of asthma. When the drug cortisone is given in large doses, it suppresses normal cortisone production by the body. This can cause atrophy of the adrenal glands so that cortisone replacement becomes a lifelong therapy. There are many other side effects and disadvantages of cortisone therapy which make its use undesirable. If auto urine therapy proves to be an effective means of supplanting exogenous cortisone, then it is a valuable adjunct to therapy.

Other people who are against urine therapy say that it is unnatural and that urine is a waste containing toxins and poisons, as well as being foul tasting and smelling. We can only say from our experience, that when one is eating a low salt, low protein (preferably vegetarian) diet, the taste of urine is not unpleasant. We have not experienced any ill effects from its use, but rather the contrary. People with a high meat intake should not use auto urine therapy, however. Seek guidance if in doubt, or if you have some other illness, especially any kidney, liver and heart disorders.

Auto-urine therapy for asthma consists of three main approaches:

1. Combined with fasting: The day before the fast eat a light meal. The next day drink most of your urine (midstream).z Between the taking of urine, drink a glass of water. You will find your urine becoming clear, copious and mild tasting. However, do not drink excessive amounts of water. If you want to fast more that twenty-four hours or if you experience hunger, you can have

57

fruit and some milk or a little vegetable broth. For one hour before and after the meal, drink no water or urine. Continue fasting if you wish.

2. Every morning drink the first flow of urine. Do not eat or drink, except water, for one hour after.

3. Massage urine into the chest, back, hands, face, head and neck. This is very relaxing.

To overcome the initial psychological distaste for urine gently rub some on your skin and smell it. Then place a small drop on your tongue, and in this way you will gradually become accustomed to it. After this, treatment becomes easy.

11

The Path to Health

Asthma attacks are generally brought about by a combination of physical and mental factors. These can result either from the person's own thinking or from his response to his relationships with other people. In addition, however, an attack of asthma can be caused simply by the fear of having it.

Through the use of yogic principles and techniques asthma attacks can be reduced and the likelihood of their recurring reduced. Some important points to remember, in terms of strengthening the mind and improving health, are:

1. Be aware when you feel that someone is making unnecessary demands on you. Of course, it is impossible not to be somewhat affected by other people's attitudes and expectations; try not to let them control your life, however.

2. Don't worry about situations which might occur in the future. Catastrophes you anticipate usually don't occur. When they do, you will muddle through somehow.

3. This applies especially to anticipated asthma attacks. Here, however, you can do something about the future right now. The yoga practices listed in this book, if faithfully carried out, will change the vicious circle of fear of an attack producing an attack, producing fear of future attacks, to the virtuous circle of confidence leading to fewer attacks, leading to more confidence.

4. The yoga practices and the general way of life recommended in this book may require a major change in your schedule and habits. This will be difficult in the beginning; overcoming old conditioning is always a test of our desire for improvement.

5. Once you have made the change and find yourself becoming healthier and more flexible, your entire attitude to life will change. Through yoga you can continue to grow, becoming physically and emotionally healthier than you dream possible.

Diabetes and Yoga

12

Diabetes Mellitus

Diabetes mellitus is a disease which has plagued man for centuries though its incidence at present, especially in the more developed areas of the world, is higher than it has ever been in the past. The reason for this is that, through technological achievement, both stress and affluence have become increasingly widespread, and people have developed the tendency to avoid strenuous physical exercise and to overeat. Thus, the recent flourishing of diabetes (and diseases which stem from the same fundamental cause) can be considered to be a side effect of the twentieth century technological age, pollution on the personal level reflecting global pollution.

At the present time modern medical science holds that there is no positive system of cure for diabetes mellitus. The most it can offer is control of the symptoms through dietary controls and daily use of insulin and other drugs. The disease itself, however, is commonly not affected by this, and may even increase in severity.

The ancient science of yoga has a more successful method of management which is thousands of years old. It is based upon the internal readjustment of the physical organism through stimulation of the body's own regenerative processes. After many years of successfully dealing with sufferers of diabetes through implementing the integral yogic system, we wish to make the knowledge of these efficacious techniques available to all interested sufferers and therapists of diabetes in the world.

Sugar metabolism

Any person undergoing yoga therapy for diabetes should know the principles involved. Diabetes mellitus is a disorder of the body's metabolism characterized by a high blood sugar level and the subsequent excretion of sugar in the urine. The human body requires sugar for energy to maintain the organs and tissues of the body. The sugar, which is taken into the body in the form of carbohydrates, enters the blood in the form of glucose (mainly), fructose and galactose. These sugars are either immediately used by the body or else are stored for later use in the liver and muscles in the form of glycogen.

When we eat a meal containing protein, carbohydrate and fat, the following things happen in the normal situation.
1. Glucose enters the bloodstream from the intestines.
2. Insulin is then released from the pancreas in order to help the glucose (from carbohydrates) and amino acids (from proteins) to be assimilated by the body.
3. Insulin pushes the glucose into skeletal muscle, fat cells and liver.
4. Fat from the meal, in the form of triglyceride, is also pushed into fat cells by insulin.

Because we do not eat continuously, periods of relative abundance alternate with food-free periods. During fasting the insulin levels reach their nadir and fat is released as a source of fuel. It is from this fat that ketones can build up to toxic levels in some people with diabetes.

The blood sugar regulates its own level. When the blood sugar level is high, the Islets of Langerhans (a group of endocrine gland cells in the pancreas with the specific function of secreting hormones) secrete insulin to lower the sugar level. The opposite effect occurs when glucagon, another Islet cell hormone, is secreted. Thus balance is achieved.

64

The regulation of sugar by the body is a very complex thing as glucose is the basic energy supplier of all body tissues. It plays an important role in all body functions and therefore requires sensitive and precise interaction of the pancreas, pituitary gland, muscles, liver, bloodstream, adrenal glands, thyroid gland, skin, kidneys and nervous system. So glucose monitoring and control is a very complex thing. It is easy to understand, therefore, why diabetes is such a complex disease and beyond the reach of medical therapy alone.

Diabetes mellitus is a chronic imbalance in the mechanism regulating blood sugar level. When it occurs, the glucose absorbed into the blood from the digestive system is prevented from being effectively used in the muscles and tissues, or from being stored in the liver in the form of glycogen or as fat. It is caused either by a relative or absolute lack of the hormone insulin.

Absolute (juvenile-onset) diabetes

In this condition for various reasons, the pancreas stops producing insulin. It can completely stop its production or it can dribble out insufficient quantities. This prevents glucose from entering the body cells, with the result that they starve, even though there is a high level of food in the form of glucose in the blood stream. This starvation affects the beta cells of the pancreas, compounding the problem and turning it into a vicious circle. This form of diabetes most commonly occurs in young people, and is a case of "Water, water everywhere, but not a drop to drink!" This form of diabetes is rarely cured, even with the use of yoga.

Relative (mature-onset) diabetes

Due to malfunction or imbalance in the nervous, hormonal and digestive systems, there is thought to be an inappropriate secretion of insulin at the wrong time, and/or the body tissues have become less responsive to insulin. In this form of diabetes, insulin release appears to occur too late in the cycle, so the blood sugar level rises to a high level before insulin is secreted. When insulin is finally liberated, there is not enough to cope with the high blood sugar level. The pancreas tries to secret more insulin, but it is too late, for by then the liver has started to release glucose in response to the call from the starving body cells. Thus the level of sugar in the blood rises even higher. In addition to this, the insulin that is released may be ineffective in letting the glucose into the cells because the cells themselves can not take it in or because insulin is poorly manufactured. There are various degrees of this type of diabetes, from mild to severe. Some cases are even unnoticeable (latent). Factors involved in mature-onset diabetes seem to be heredity, increasing age, obesity, infections and stress.

Symptoms of diabetes

The high blood glucose concentration causes more glucose to pass through the kidneys, drawing out with it large quantities of water. This results in:

• Excessive urine with a high glucose content
• Excessive thirst
• Dehydration
• Excess glucose in all body fluids, supplying food for bacteria, making one more prone to infections. For instance, simple wounds tend to fester badly.

The cells, in order to keep alive, start using fat as a fuel instead of glucose. This produces an added penalty in the form of fatty acids (called ketones) in the tissues. As a result, the patient develops severe acidosis. This, in association with dehydration, can cause diabetic coma (unconsciousness). Death may result unless the condition is treated immediately with the appropriate doses of insulin.

The more advanced a case of diabetes, the more extreme symptoms will become. Mature-onset diabetes occurs predominantly in affluent middle-aged persons who are abnormally obese. It is due to a relative lack of insulin. This stems from the fact the diet is generally heavy in sugar-rich carbohydrates, and this is often combined with insufficient exercise to work off the large amounts of glucose which are consumed.

It is our belief that many persons who now suffer from mature-onset diabetes could have completely avoided the disease if they had limited their intake of sugar-rich carbohydrates to a reasonable level and participated in a modicum of daily exercise, preferably yogic in nature. The daily practice of meditation would also have helped to reduce the chance of contracting diabetes by establishing balance in the nervous system, thereby not allowing the body to become out of tune with itself.

It is with mature-onset diabetes that we are mainly concerned. It affects the larger proportion of diabetics, and is potentially reversible. Juvenile diabetes with absolute lack of insulin can also be greatly helped through yoga, though its reversal is rare. Yoga can help prevent the complications of juvenile-onset diabetes.

All diabetics are encouraged to take up yoga so that they may gain increased health through this science. All can benefit, depending on how much effort is put into the practice. The longer you have had diabetes, the more effort you will require. A positive attitude and persistent practice of the correct techniques over a long period will pay valuable dividends, even in the severest case of diabetes.

At the Bihar School of Yoga, we have had most success in treating mature-onset diabetes when it is first detected. Even a young person who has just discovered he has high blood sugar levels has a good chance of eradicating the problem. Unfortunately, most people do not come to yoga until they realize that medicines are no answer to their disease. This is an important point to remember. Combinations of medicines and yoga are the best way to attack diabetic problems, especially before it becomes set into the body.

13

Importance of Correct Insulin Dosage

W e are including this list of the signs and symptoms of hyper and hypoglycaemia to enable the team of doctor, yoga teacher and student to regulate the student's dosage of insulin while he/she is adjusting to the new diet and the practices involved in the diabetic training program.

Hyperglycaemia

This is a sign of diabetes that every patient will recognize as it occurred before treatment started. The symptoms are: excessive thirst and hunger; excessive urination; the need to go to the toilet many times during the night; tiredness; loss of weight; white marks on the clothing; itching around the vulva or the penis; increasing short-sightedness; loss of the sensation of pain in the limbs; impotence.

There is a much controversy as to whether insulin injections help to prevent these symptoms: failing vision; loss of sensation or pain in the limbs; infection of the skin, lungs or urinary tract; impotence. It is up to the patient, yoga therapist and doctor to decide what steps to take if symptoms persist and health deteriorates. Infections must be treated medically, but conditions should not deter the team from continuing the practice program. Modern medicine has still not been able to find solutions to these problems.

If the following symptoms of keto-acidosis occur, insulin is required immediately and a doctor and ambulance will be

68

needed at once. The symptoms are: pain in the upper abdomen; vomiting; intense thirst and excessive urination; constipation; altered vision; muscle cramps. Physical signs are dry tongue and soft eyeballs due to dehydration; deep sighing respiration; a rapid, weak pulse; low blood pressure; abdominal rigidity and tenderness; coma. No diabetic who has used insulin for some time would allow himself to get to this stage, so the symptoms are listed here only as a general precaution.

Any acute infection may lead to keto-acidosis and therefore every infection must be treated under the supervision of a doctor. Remember that any form of infection or stress can precipitate this condition even in the case of mild diabetes. The most common cause is neglect of treatment due to carelessness, misunderstanding or illness, or failure to adjust the treatment in the event of acute infection.

Hypoglycaemia

If you take too much insulin your blood glucose level will drop and a dangerous condition called hypoglycaemia can occur. When you are using yogic practices which increase the body's own insulin or reduce the blood glucose you must keep a close watch on the blood glucose level. This is why we recommend the following:

1. Kidney tests to check kidney function – by this we mean the level of sugar, protein, blood and so on in the urine, and other tests such as serum creatinine. Other tests, such as an IVP, can also be done if thought necessary by your doctor.

2. Regular blood glucose tests – at least once a week until you restabilize. Compare the results of this test with urine glucose tests to ensure that the glucose levels in the urine faithfully reflect those in the blood. Sometimes, if diabetes affects the kidneys, the urine sugar level is high which seems to reflect a high blood sugar level. This is a misleading situation which may cause us to take more insulin than we need, thus precipitating hypoglycaemia.

Tests must also be compared from time to time in case there is a reversal in the condition of the kidneys.

3. Urine tests at least daily – carried out according to your doctor's instructions.
4. Watch for symptoms of hypoglycaemia – this should also be done by the people around you. The symptoms of hypoglycaemia (too much insulin and too little sugar) are as follows:
   a) *Early*: weakness, hunger, sweating, heart palpitations, tremor (shaking)
   b) *Later* : dizziness, confusion, unsteadiness
   c) *Advanced*: drunken appearance, mental confusion, slurring speech, staggering, imbalance, wanting to sleep
   d) *Very advanced*: unconsciousness (coma).

The remedy for hypoglycaemia is simple – eat some pure glucose. Therefore, always keep some handy in your pocket, in the form of small sweets. The consequences of not doing this can be fatal. It is always better to have a little more than a little less sugar in the blood.

If there is no response within ten minutes to the ingestion of some pure glucose in the case of suspected hypoglycaemia, the diabetic should go to the nearest hospital, or doctor if the hospital is too far away.

Conclusion

It has been a rare thing in our experience for the problems of hyper or hypoglycaemia to cause any inconvenience to the diabetic yoga practitioner who is normally aware of his condition and the possible complications. Most diabetics have experienced both ends of the spectrum at one time or another, and will advise those in charge of their treatment on how to meet these situations. The patient himself is the most sensitive monitor of his treatment. If this is kept clearly in mind, there should be no difficulties in combining yogic management with medical treatment, and the person will be well on the way to a more healthy and free existence.

14

Diabetes and Diet

The subject of what diabetics should eat is best dealt with by a dietician. However, from the practical point of view, we have found that there are certain foods that are beneficial for diabetics, especially when combined with a yoga program. It is known that dietary compliance is seldom good, so dietary prescription should not be too rigid and should be individualized for the patient's culture, type of disease, etc. Diet is more important for non-insulin dependent diabetes than for insulin treated patients in whom any extra stress of the diet is dealt with by a little extra insulin.

All nutritionists will agree that for good health a variety of minimally processed foods with lots of fresh nutrients and fibre is best. Research has found that insulin dosage can often be reduced with a high fibre diet, such as whole grains, beans and vegetables – an ashram diet. It is also known that, as diabetics have an increased incidence of heart disease and high blood pressure, moderate weight loss alone combined with exercise will bring about a general improvement. Many people have stopped using anti-diabetic drugs following the combination of a yogic lifestyle and diet.

The diet should be low fat because high fat diets impair carbohydrate metabolism and increase the chances of getting heart disease. The American Diabetic Association recommends a diet in which 60–70% of calories come from carbohydrates, while the rest of the diet should be 20–30%

71

protein and 10–20% fats. Whatever fats are taken into the body should be unsaturated (usually plant and vegetable origin) rather than saturated fats (animal origin).

As a general dictum for diabetes avoid excess amounts of simple sugars, such as white sugar, honey, glucose and other forms of sweets. Eat more complex carbohydrates such as wheat, oatmeal, buckwheat, corn and wholegrain (unrefined) rice. Also salt intake should be low and alcohol no more than moderate. However, research shows that diabetics may be able to occasionally eat a minimal amount of sugar. It is important to follow your doctor's guidelines in this matter and a good doctor who is up on the latest research will advise you accordingly to your individual needs. However, as a general guideline the following is a good diabetic and general health diet:

1. *Vegetables (group A)*: the following vegetables contain insignificant carbohydrates and calories. As a salad, you can eat as much as you like. When cooked, the intake should be limited to about one quarter litre of cooked vegetables (boiled, baked or steamed, not fried), e.g. cabbage, cauliflower, cucumber, eggplant (brinjal), spinach, okra (lady's fingers), tomato, parwal (gourd), celery, bitter gourd (karela).

2. *Vegetables (group B)*: each portion contains approximately 14 grams of carbohydrate and 4 grams of protein (about 80 calories) per measuring cup (¼ litre), e.g. carrots, onions, green peas.

3. *Fruits*: each portion contains 10 grams of carbohydrate (approximately 40 calories) for each item mentioned: 1 orange, 1 guava, ⅓ papaya, ½ apple, ½ banana, 1 cup water melon.

4. *Cereals*: each portion contains 25 grams of carbohydrate and 2 grams of protein (approximately 70 calories) for each item mentioned: 2 and ½ tablespoons of wheat, jawar, millet (bajara) or corn flour, ½ cup of cooked rice or khichari (rice cooked with lentils), 20 grams of non-sweetened biscuits, 100 grams of boiled potato.

5. *Pulses*: as a rule, 1 cup (1 portion of cooked dal (pulses), e.g. lentils, mung beans, split peas) contains approximately 140 calories.
6. *Fats*: one portion contains 5 grams of fat (approximately 50 calories) for each item: 1 teaspoon butter, oil or ghee; 10 grams of cashew nuts, ground nuts or almonds.
7. *Milk*: each portion supplies 12 grams of carbohydrate, 8 grams of protein, 10 grams of fat (approximately 170 calories) per item: ¼ litre whole milk (1 cup), 1 cup yoghurt, 240 grams each.

On this basis a typical diabetic diet would be as follows (the numbers indicate how many portions):
- *Breakfast*: 1 bread + 1 milk + 1 fruit + 1 fat or a handful of sprouted mung beans.
- *Lunch*: 1 vegetable (group A) + 1 vegetable (group B) + 3 cereal + 2 pulse + 3 fat + ½ yoghurt + 1 fruit.
- *Tea*: ½ milk + 1 bread, or 1 fruit + 10 grams nuts.
- *Dinner*: 1 vegetable (group A) + 1 vegetable (group B) + 3 cereal + 1 pulse + 2 fat + 1 fruit.
- *Bedtime*: ⅓ milk or 2 fruits.

This example of a diabetic diet should supply approximately 2000 to 2500 calories per day and should be adjusted to suit your needs and wants by a skilled professional, e.g. you may need more calories during heavy exercise.

When this diet is combined with a yogic sadhana, and once the blood sugar has been controlled by a combination of yoga, diet and medicines as required, the diet can be readjusted. However, this kind of diet is very close to the one used in the ashram and is recommended for most people as a light, balanced diet which should enhance general health and increase the lifespan.

Both patient and doctor should not only be aware of the wide variety of good and tasty foods available to the diabetic, but also that it is the addition of yoga that can transform the life of the patient, increasing awareness of needs and capacity, promoting digestion and metabolism and offering the reward of new health, vitality and a higher consciousness.

15

Yogic Treatment of Diabetes

Meditation

The mind, through the nervous system, controls every action and reaction that occurs in the human body. It keeps a record of everything that a person and his body have undergone in the past and relates it to the present conditions. From this function come the decisions which rule every action that a person makes, whether voluntary or involuntary. This control extends from the unconscious and automatic control of the organs and muscles right up to the decisions that are made with the conscious intellectual mind. Every person's whole existence is based upon the correct function of the nervous system.

The science of yoga holds that the nervous system (and the body that it rules) can be brought under a high degree of control and can be made to operate with the greatest possible degree of efficiency through the practice of meditation. This ancient theory has been bolstered by scientific research done in India, Europe and the United States. The bulk of this research has shown conclusively that the daily practice of meditation brings about harmonious changes in the physical organism.

In regard to diabetes, meditation practices have been shown definitely to help the endocrine glands through relaxation of the sympathetic nervous system arising from practices such as ajapa japa. Regulation of the anterior pituitary hormones, which are under the direct control of the hypothalamus, is greatly affected by yoga nidra. Also, a general increase in mental efficiency is brought about.

Hatha yoga

Of equal importance in the treatment of diabetes are the hatha yoga practices of shankhaprakshalana and kunjal kriya. Shankhaprakshalana is the systematic cleansing of the alimentary tract, which runs from the mouth to the anus. In this kriya a large amount of warm saline water is ingested, two glasses at a time, alternated with five special asanas. These asanas open the sphincter muscles, which control digestive motions and move the water rapidly down the alimentary canal. After a few glasses, the practitioner automatically starts to go to the latrine to pass the water mixed with the former contents of the stomach and intestines.

By the end of the practice the whole digestive system has been flushed out and pure water is being passed. After this is completed, the practitioner rests totally for forty-five to sixty minutes. This period is the only opportunity that the digestive system (including the pancreas and liver) ever gets to really rest, because only when the intestines are completely empty, do digestive nerve impulses and glandular secretions stop. In this short time, the internal organs are able to revitalize themselves and when the rest period is finished the practitioner eats a simple meal of khichari (rice boiled with lentils and ghee). This allows the system to start up again in the easiest and most balanced way. Shankhaprakshalana is then continued in its brief form (laghoo shankhaprakshalana) every day for 40 days, and during this time the blood sugar level of even serious sufferers of diabetes often drops to normal, or close to normal, and can remain there indefinitely unless the system is again thrown out of balance. Therefore, it is important to monitor the blood sugar levels regularly during this time so that medication can be adjusted following the yoga practices.

Asana and pranayama

In conjunction with meditation and shankhaprakshalana, a series of asanas and pranayama is to be practised in the treatment of diabetes. These asanas adjust the function of the organs involved by regulating nervous impulses and blood flow to the glandular areas and by gently massaging all the glands and organs. Pranayama controls the body's energy, allowing vital forces to flow to those areas that require extra energy. The brain, pancreas and other organs can then be revitalized consciously and systematically.

16

Course Program

The following therapeutic practice programs have been found to be very useful in the treatment of diabetes and for strengthening the body and mind. Yoga practices have powerful effects, bringing about subtle and profound changes in the body and mind. Therefore, they should be chosen appropriately and practised properly. Otherwise the desired effect will not be achieved and under some circumstances there may be an adverse effect. A yoga therapy program should be individually prescribed for each person and supervised by a qualified yoga teacher. At the same time the practices themselves should be learnt correctly and practised in a relaxed manner.

The yoga programs outlined here are in 3 stages, with each consecutive stage including more advanced practices. At least 3 months is recommended for each stage, and that can be considerably extended according to individual needs. You should move on to the next stage of the program only after having done all the practices from the previous stage with ease, without any physical or mental strain, for a period of at least one month. This will ensure the greatest therapeutic benefits. As your familiarity with the practices grows, you will be able to adjust the program according to your needs. In stages 2 and 3, practices from the first stage can continue to be incorporated. Their value and effect should not be overlooked. You will find that the yoga practices are not difficult to do. Given the time and necessary effort they require, you will find yourself richly rewarded by the beneficial changes they can bring about.

These therapy programs address those people who have uncomplicated diabetes, that is without any associated disorders, such as high blood pressure or heart disease. If you have any other medical problems apart from diabetes, you should consult a qualified yoga therapist for proper guidance before starting. That is the safest and fastest way. However, all the practices in stage one, if done in the correct way, have been found to be safe in nearly all circumstances. Check the contra-indications for all the practices where necessary and consult your yoga therapist. As the effects of the yoga practices build up, blood sugar levels can drop significantly.

Remember: The treatment of diabetes through yoga is an involved, technical process. The management of diabetes should not be attempted without the direct guidance of an experienced yoga teacher. All practices should be learnt correctly from a yoga teacher. The programs and practices given here should act as guidelines only.

Please also read the introduction in the 'Practices' section.

Stage 1: Long program
Jala neti: daily.

Laghoo shankhaprakshalana (start after 1 month): twice a week for one month, then once a week.

Tadasana: 3 rounds.

Trikonasana (start with variation 3, then gradually move into variation 1 and 2): 3 rounds.

Utthita lolasana: 5 rounds.

Kati chakrasana: 5 rounds.

Pawanmuktasana part 1 – practices for legs, arms and neck on alternating days: 6–10 rounds.

Pawanmuktasana part 2 – go through the whole series by practising two practices at a time, for a minimum period of 3 weeks: 3–8 rounds.

Marjari-asana: 5–8 rounds.
Bhujangasana: 3 rounds.
Shashankasana: 3 rounds, rest in final position of last round
    for 10–27 abdominal breaths.
Meru wakrasana: 5 rounds.
Abdominal breathing: 11 rounds.
Yogic breathing in shavasana: 27 rounds.
Nadi shodhana, techniques 1 and 2 – 1:1. Start with com-
    fortable count, gradually extend up to 10:10 – 5 rounds.
Bhramari: 9 rounds.
Moola bandha: 10 rounds.
Relaxation/yoga nidra.

Stage 1: Short program
Tadasana: 3 rounds.
Pawanmuktasana part 1: 3 practices per day; go systemati-
    cally through the whole series.
Marjari-asana: 5 rounds.
Bhujangasana: 3 rounds.
Shashankasana static: for 11 breaths.
Abdominal and yogic breathing: 11 rounds each. After 1
    month replace with nadi shodhana, techniques 1 and 2 –
    1:1, gradually extend count to 10:10 – 5 rounds.
Bhramari: 9 rounds.
Relaxation/yoga nidra.
Shatkarmas: as in long program.

Stage 2: Long program
Jala neti: on alternating days.
Laghoo shankhaprakshalana and kunjal (with jala neti) –
    twice a week for one month, then once a week.
Surya namaskara: 3–5 rounds.
Shavasana with abdominal breathing until heart beat and
    breath return to normal.
Shashank bhujangasana: 5 rounds.
Naukasana: 3 rounds.
Tadagi mudra: 3 rounds x 10.

Gomukhasana: 1 round each side, gradually extend length of time in final position.

Ardha matsyendrasana (easy variation): 1 round each side

Vipareeta karani asana: 10 seconds to 1 minute.

Matsyasana (lying on the back): half time as in vipareeta karani asana.

Agnisar kriya (start with swana pranayama, after one month move on to actual kriya), 10–20 breaths: 3–5 rounds.

Nadi shodhana technique 2, 1:2, gradually build up to technique 3, 1:1:1 – 5 rounds.

Bhramari: 9 rounds, or ujjayi: 5 minutes.

Moola bandha, technique 2, with internal breath retention: 5 rounds.

Yoga nidra/relaxation.

Ajapa japa, technique 1 (frontal passage, stages 1, 2 and 3): one month of each stage: 10–15 minutes in the evening.

Stage 2: Short program

Shatkarmas: as in stage 2 long program.

Shashshank bhujangasana: 5 rounds.

Naukasana: 3 rounds.

Tadagi mudra 3 rounds for 10.

Gomukhasana: 1 round each side.

Meru wakrasana: 5 rounds.

Agnisar kriya: as in stage 2 long version.

Nadi shodhana: as in stage 2 long version.

Ajapa japa: as in stage 2 long version.

Stage 3

Shatkarmas, same as in stage 2, or can be adjusted to suit the needs of the practitioner.

Jala neti: twice a week.

Laghoo shankhaprakshalana and kunjal: once a week or once in 15 days, depending on the condition of the practitioner.

Poorna shankhaprakshalana, under expert guidance, if conditions permit.

Surya namaskara: 5 rounds.

Shavasana with abdominal breathing: 27 breaths.

Pawanmuktasana part 2.

Supta udarakarshanasana: 5 rounds.

Dhanurasana: 3 rounds, gradually extend time in final position and reduce to one round only.

Paschimottanasana: 3 rounds.

Sarvangasana/vipareeta karani asana (depending on flexibility): 10 seconds–1 minute.

Matsyasana: half the time spent in sarvangasana/vipareeta karani asana.

Yogamudrasana: as long as matsyasana.

Gomukhasana: one round each side.

Ardha matsyendrasana: one round each side, gradually extend time in final position.

Bhastrika: 3–5 rounds, 20 breaths. In the second month introduce jalandhara and moola bandha at the end of each round.

Nadi shodhana, technique 3, 1:1:2, eventually extending to 1:2:2 – 5 rounds.

Bhramari: 9 rounds, or ujjayi: 5 minutes.

Yoga nidra/relaxation.

Ajapa japa, technique 2 (spinal passage, stages 1,2 and 3): one month of each stage: 10–20 minutes in the evening.

17

Low Blood Sugar

Low blood sugar, or reactive hypoglycaemia, is a common condition. It seems likely that more people suffer from this condition than high blood sugar, though present-day figures are unreliable because of the vague nature of the condition and the fact that it often goes undiagnosed. It is even possible that the majority of people today suffer from it in mild form and thereby feel tired and exhausted and the need for a pick-up, such as a cup of coffee.

Symptoms

The most common features of true hypoglycaemia are a feeling of tiredness, depression and irritability, wanting to be left alone. Other symptoms include a hollow empty feeling, headaches, poor concentration, forgetfulness and vague spells. Most people suffer from more than one of these symptoms, which tend to be periodic, occurring mainly first thing in the morning, mid-morning (around 11 a.m.) and mid-afternoon (between 3 and 4 p.m.) and between 2 and 3 a.m. Symptoms are relieved sometimes within just a few minutes, by eating. A good symptom-free period after dinner is also a feature.

All of us experience the cyclic fluctuation of hormones, energy, body rhythms, moods, emotions and thoughts, throughout the day, and some people are more stable than others. The person with hypoglycaemia, however, experiences sometimes violent or distressing fluctuations between high and low energy states which are difficult to explain. Even doctors may not appreciate, at first, what is going on. The symptoms of hypoglycaemia are caused by instability of the glucose regulating mechanisms of the body so that a few hours after eating the blood sugar drops to low levels, below most maintained for fasting in normal people. This low blood sugar level affects the metabolism and energy level and the above symptoms arise.

Causes

Some of the main causes of this problem are: chronic stress, which disturbs the brain's controlling systems and manifests as autonomic nervous system, endocrine and metabolic imbalance; lack of exercise; and, perhaps most important, the excessive consumption of sugar and refined carbohydrates.

There are certain foods which the body cannot deal with properly and these are especially refined and junk foods. Many Western diets are characterized by the excessive consumption of processed, over-refined foods which may contain large quantities of simple sugars, for example, sucrose (white and brown table sugar), white flour, white rice, white bread, biscuits, cakes, instant and canned foods, packaged breakfast cereals, and so on.

The sugar problem

The consumption of sugar today has increased greatly as more and more sugar becomes available and is added into different preparations. One hundred years ago we ate one kilogram of precious sugar every few months. However, today the average person consumes approximately one kilogram of sugar per week, and most of this is hidden in foods. If we think about it, we eat a lot of sugar in coffee, tea, cereals, sweets, cakes, chocolate, jam, milk, yoghurt and also in the form of honey and other sweeteners. If we also take snacks between meals, the average consumption of sugar may rise to double or more.

We may ask, what is so wrong with the sugar anyway? There are two points to remember in terms of why sugar in excess is bad for us.

1. Most forms of sugar, except honey and raw unprocessed sugar straight from the sugar cane, and most refined foods are devoid of any real nutritional value. They usually contain a lot of calories, however, and thereby tend to increase body weight and fat storage without contributing any of the vitamins and minerals so necessary for good health, fitness and well-being.

2. Eating simple, processed sugar (as opposed to complex sugars found in wholegrain wheat, rice and so on), strains and causes an imbalance of the sugar regulating mechanisms of the body. Each time we eat simple sugar, it is quickly absorbed into the body, provoking a rapid and intense insulin secretion in order to cope with the large amount of blood sugar. If this is repeated several times each day for many years, the pancreas and neural regulating mechanisms may become imbalanced resulting in either high or low blood sugar.

High blood sugar, diabetes, may result when the pancreas and nerves become fatigued and either cannot produce enough insulin or release the insulin too late.

Low blood sugar occurs when we eat a highly sugared meal. The blood sugar level rises quickly causing the pancreas to over-react and over-secrete insulin so that the sugar level falls to very low levels. The brain starves, thereby producing symptoms of fatigue and exhaustion. Initially the intake of simple sugar gives us a quick burst of energy, a high. However, this quickly runs down and we soon feel weak, depressed, unable to concentrate. This pushes us to seek new highs through stimulants such as coffee, tea and other sugar filled foods, and so the vicious circle goes on.

Because the condition is vague and non-specific, it is not readily diagnosed unless special blood tests are performed and a busy doctor may dismiss the condition as psychogenic (mental), neurotic or hypochondriacal.

What to do?

The first step in overcoming hypoglycaemia is to stop eating processed, refined and junk foods and reduce sugar intake. Sugar or honey can be taken once or twice per day in small doses as long as the rest of the diet is good and yoga practices are performed. Otherwise a doctor will advise complete cession of the sugar intake.

The diet should include whole grains, pulses (lentils and dal), plenty of fresh vegetables both raw and cooked, whole nuts, sprouted mung beans or chickpeas (channa). Wheat is usually preferable to rice and other starchy food. Oil, ghee, fried food and spices should be kept to an absolute minimum as they cause sluggishness of the digestion and metabolism. A moderate, balanced intake of milk products and fruits should also be eaten.

Sometimes a vitamin and mineral supplement containing B group multivitamins, vitamin C (500 mg per day) and a balance of minerals such as calcium, zinc, magnesium, chromium, manganese and selenium is required.

Practices

18

Introduction

Of the many yogic practices in common use, only those most relevant to the specific needs of people suffering from asthma and diabetes are included here. The selection has been made with a view to alleviating the physical and mental problems associated with these illnesses, improving general health and as a beginning on the path of spirituality. Further practices are included in *Asana Pranayama Mudra Bandha*, published by Yoga Publications Trust. Although all the techniques in this book are fully and clearly explained for home practice, no book can replace the insight and experience of a trained yoga teacher. Personal instruction from an experienced teacher is essential for curing disease in the quickest, safest and most efficient way. If you do not heed this advice, you are taking unnecessary risks with your health.

For further guidance in finding a qualified teacher please contact:

Bihar School of Yoga, Munger 811201, Bihar, India
Email: bsy@yogavision.net
Website: www.yogavision.net

Before practising

During episodes of illnesses like common cold, flu, seasonal fever, dysentery or any other acute short-term illness, you should discontinue all practices except shavasana and yoga nidra, and resume your program only after full recovery has been achieved. If the illness lasts for a week or more, when you resume your daily yogic practices, you should go back one step and start with the stage previous to the one you had been doing before the illness, and then gradually build up from there.

As the effects of yoga therapy build up and your condition improves, the necessity for medication is reduced, and appropriate adjustment – reduction in doses of medicines – may be needed, to avoid a possibility of an overdose. Periodical medical check-ups by your doctor should be done on a regular basis. This applies particularly to people suffering from diabetes who are on insulin, in order to avoid potentially dangerous attacks of hypoglycaemia, if the insulin dose is not suitably adjusted. This should be done only under strict medical guidance.

Ideal times for practising
Asana, pranayama, mudra and bandha are best practised in the morning before breakfast. The next best time is before the evening meal, after a short period of relaxation. Late morning before lunch is another alternative.

Meditation, in particular, and yoga nidra are most effective when practised in the evening: yoga nidra early in the evening, and meditation before going to sleep.

Yoga nidra, even a short practice, at some time in the day, is highly recommended if the time can be found.

19

Cleansing Practices

The hatha yoga shatkarmas consist of six practices of purification that remove toxins from the body and mind. These exercises are very important from the point of view of health and longevity. The physical body only wears out at the average age of seventy years because we are constantly accumulating toxins and impurities in the body systems and our habits and daily actions do not give the body the chance to remove them. These impurities decrease our reserves of energy and good health. However, this can be reduced by adopting the habitual practice of yogic cleansing techniques.

The six cleansing kriyas are dhauti, basti, neti, nauli, trataka and kapalbhati, but included here are only those practices that are most specific and useful to asthma and diabetes. They are sufficient to purify the body and mind and to start you on the path to good health. Once this process begins, it continues unaided as an ongoing cycle of good health.

The practices of shatkarma outlined in this section should be learned from and practised under the guidance of an experienced yoga teacher. For complete details of the practices outlined consult the relevant chapter on shatkarma in *Asana Pranayama Mudra Bandha* published by Yoga Publications Trust.

Kunjal kriya (the practice of vomiting water)

Preparation: Take some lukewarm water, enough for approximately six glasses (2 litres) per person and add salt, at the ratio of one teaspoon per litre of water – (more salt can be added if necessary). Mix the water and salt thoroughly.

Technique: Drink at least six glasses of the prepared salt water one after another as quickly as possible while standing.

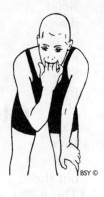

Immediately after drinking the six glasses lean forward and place the middle and index fingers of the right hand as far back in the throat as possible. The fingernails should be short and clean.

Rub and press the back of the tongue. This will induce a strong urge to vomit and the water will be thrown out of the mouth in a series of quick gushes.

Press the tongue until the stomach is empty.

Time of practice: Early in the morning with an empty stomach. Kunjal should also be performed after completing the practice of shankhaprakshalana.

Precautions: Wait for at least twenty minutes before eating food after doing this practice.

Contra-indications: Kunjal should not be practised by people with high blood pressure, heart disease, stroke, ulcer, hernia or diabetes with eye problems.

Jala neti (nasal cleansing with water)

Preparation: A special vessel called a neti lota is used (see diagram). If this type of vessel is not available, use a teapot with a small spout.

Fill the vessel with pure, lukewarm water, at blood temperature, suitable for pouring into the nose.

Add salt, about one teaspoonful per litre of water, making sure it is completely dissolved.

Stage 1: Washing the nostrils

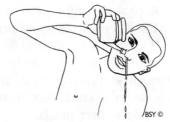

Bend forward with the face down and insert the spout of the lota gently into the left nostril.

Slowly tilt the head to the right, while simultaneously elevating the lota in such a way that water runs into the left nostril.

Breathe through the open mouth.

The water should flow through the left nostril and then out through the right nostril.

This will happen automatically, providing the position of the lota and the angle of the head are correct, and the respiration is through the open mouth.

Allow the water to flow freely through the nostrils for about twenty seconds.

Then remove the lota and clean the nose by blowing through the nostrils.

Do not blow too hard; the practitioner should use discretion in this respect, taking care not to put pressure on the ears.

Repeat the same process, pouring the water into the right nostril and tilting the head to the left. After completion, repeat once again through the left nostril and finally again through the right nostril.

Stage 2: Drying the nostrils

Stand erect with feet together. Clasp the hands behind the back. Bend forward from the waist and let the head hang. Remain in this position for about thirty seconds.

This will allow all the water to drain from the nose.

Then, while in the stooping position, blow through the nose five times. Then stand erect again.

Close one of the nostrils by gently pressing the side of that nostril with one finger.

Breathe in and out vigorously thirty times in quick succession, emphasizing the exhalation, as in kapalbhati pranayama, to exhaust the maximum amount of moisture. Repeat the same process with the other nostril.

Then repeat the same process with both nostrils open.

If water still remains in the nose, repeat the drying process until the nose is completely dry.

Frequency: Practise every morning, or more often in the case of a cold. Neti can be practised anytime except straight after meals.

Precautions: The water should only pass through the nose. If any water enters the throat or mouth, it indicates that the position of the head is incorrect and you should adjust the head until the water flows through the nose only. If this problem persists, consult a yoga teacher. Make sure the nose is properly dried after doing jala neti, otherwise the nasal passages may become irritated and manifest the uncomfortable symptoms of a cold. Do not blow the nose too hard.

Contra-indications: People suffering from chronic nasal bleeding should not do jala neti without expert advice.

Sutra neti (nasal cleaning with thread)

Preparation: Sutra means thread or string. Instead of the traditional string, a rubber catheter is used today and is available from most pharmacies.

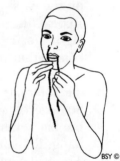

Technique: The catheter is passed through one nostril and pulled out through the mouth.

Then the catheter is pulled to and fro so that it slides backwards and forwards in the nostril.

Do this about thirty to fifty times.

Breathe in and out through the mouth.

Remove the catheter from the nostril and repeat on the other side.

Perform this after jala neti and repeat jala neti on completion of sutra neti.

Precautions: It is necessary to start under expert guidance. Do this exercise gently and slowly.

Contra-indications: Sutra neti should not be practised if there is chronic bleeding in the nose. If there is a congenital blockage of the nose, you should first seek medical advice.

Shankhaprakshalana (washing of the intestines)

Preparation: This practice should only be done under the guidance of an experienced yoga teacher. The season and day of practice should be mild and dry, neither too hot nor too cold.

The night before undertaking the practice, take only a light semi-liquid meal.

On the day of performing shankhaprakshalana no food, tea, coffee, etc. should be consumed prior to commencement of the practice.

A clean bucket or similar container should be filled with lukewarm water. Some salt must be added to the water, just enough so that the water tastes salty (about one teaspoon per litre of water).

The practices should be done in a light-hearted atmosphere and in a relaxed manner. For this reason it is best done in a group of five to ten people.

Complete intestinal wash: Drink two glasses of salty water as quickly as you can.

Then perform the following five asanas eight times each: tadasana, tiryaka tadasana, kati chakrasana, tiryaka bhujangasana and udarakarshanasana.

All the practices should be done at a steady pace in quick succession. Do not rest between rounds.

Drink two more glasses of salty water and repeat all five asanas again eight times each.

Drink two more glasses and perform the five asanas eight times each a third time.

After the third time, go to the toilet and try to evacuate the bowels.

Relax, do not strain.

If evacuation occurs or not, it does not matter; there is plenty of time.

After a minute or so in the toilet, come out and drink two more glasses.

Continue this process: drink two glasses of salty water then do the asanas eight times each. Go to the toilet. Eventually some kind of motion will occur. Do not compare yourself with the other people doing shankha-prakshalana. Some will have a quick evacuation; some will take much longer.

Do not worry if you take a longer time or if you drink more glasses than the others.

At first solid stool will start to be evacuated and then water and stool mixed. Carry on drinking water, doing the five asanas and sitting on the toilet.

Eventually the water that you pass will be clean. On an average, between sixteen and twenty glasses of salty water must be consumed before clean water is evacuated. Some people will take less and some will take more.

It is important to stop the practice when the water becomes almost clear as the system may start producing bile indicated by bright yellow water.

Supplementary practices: Shankhaprakshalana washes the region of the alimentary canal from the mouth to the anus. For perfect cleanliness of the entire digestive tract, the following two techniques should be done immediately after completing shankhaprakshalana:

Kunjal kriya: to clean the area from the stomach to the mouth and to remove any further salty water from the stomach.

Jala neti: to clean the nasal passages.

Rest: Total rest is essential. Lie down or sit quietly for exactly forty-five minutes keeping the body warm. It is important that you do not sleep. During this period of time the whole digestive system is being completely rested and revitalized.

Special food: A special food should be eaten forty-five minutes after the completion of shankhaprakshalana.

This food is a special preparation of rice, pulse (mung dal) or lentils, cooked with ghee (clarified butter). This special food is necessary to activate and lubricate the digestive tract in a gentle manner. Correct knowledge of how to prepare this food is important.

Shankhaprakshalana has removed not only all the waste from the alimentary canal, but also all the natural and absolutely necessary protective layers from the canal walls. The ghee is essential to provide a temporary protective coating until the body provides a new layer. It is not normal for the intestines to be completely empty so the rice supplies a simple digestible 'packing' material. The pulses or lentils supply a high protein food, yet one that is easy to digest. It supplements the carbohydrates in the rice and the fat from the ghee to provide a balanced meal.

Further rest and second meal: After eating further rest is necessary for the remainder of the day.

Do not sleep for three hours after the first meal.

Also take only the khichari for the next meal six hours later.

Frequency: Not more than every six months, as directed an experienced yoga teacher.

Food restrictions: These are necessary for at least a week, longer if possible.

Chemically processed, non-vegetarian and acidic foods should be strictly avoided for at least one week. Milk, buttermilk and acidic fruits such as lemons, grapefruit, oranges, etc. are also restricted.

Alcohol, cigarettes, tea, coffee, betel nut preparations such as pan should not be taken for at least a week.

The diet should be as pure, simple and neutral (not too acidic) as possible.

Remember, the whole digestive system has been cleaned and a sudden intake of toxic, poisonous and difficult to digest foods could produce bad reactions such as fever, indigestion, constipation and so on.

Contra-indications and precautions: It is very important only to attempt this practice under expert supervision. If you suffer from **any** medical condition, you should seek further guidance first.

All the guidelines and restrictions should be strictly followed.

Practice note: There are a number of sphincters or valves in the alimentary canal between the stomach and the anus, which open and close to allow the controlled passage of food during the digestive process. The five asanas which are practised during shankhaprakshalana work together to relax the muscles of these valves and allow the salty water to pass freely and quickly to the anus for discharge.

Laghoo Shankhaprakshalana (short intestinal wash)

This is the shorter version of the full practice of shankhaprakshalana.

Early in the morning before eating or drinking anything, prepare water as described for shankhaprakshalana.

Drink two glasses of salty water, and then practise the same five asanas eight times each, as described for shankhaprakshalana.

Then drink another two glasses of salty water and repeat the five asanas.

Then again drink two more glasses of salty water and repeat the asanas. You have now taken six glasses of water. This completes the practice; now you should go to the toilet.

Usually after this practice, there is a full bowel movement plus a large quantity of urine.

Additional practices: Kunjal kriya and jala neti may be performed after completing the practice.

Time of practice: This practice should be done early in the morning on an empty stomach.

Frequency: For therapeutic purposes, it may be practised daily for a limited period of time under expert supervision. Otherwise practising once or twice a week is sufficient.

Rest: On completion of the practice rest for half an hour before taking food or drink.

Restrictions: For this practice there are no diet restrictions, but common sense suggests keeping the diet as balanced as possible.

Contra-indications: As for shankhaprakshalana.

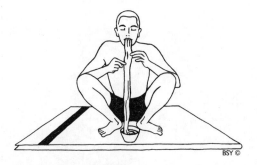

Vastra Dhauti (cloth cleansing)

Preparation: In this practice a specially prepared cloth of fine cotton about two inches wide and several feet long is used to clean the stomach.

This practice should only be performed on a completely empty stomach.

Technique: Put one end of the cloth into your mouth.

Moisten well with saliva in your mouth before swallowing the cloth.

Carefully and slowly swallow it in the same way as you would food.

You should drink a little water every minute or so to make the cloth go down more easily.

Don't swallow all the cloth. Hold one end loose so that it can eventually be withdrawn.

Keep the cloth in the stomach for some time, but no longer than twenty minutes.

If you know nauli or agnisar kriya you should perform them.

Then gently withdraw the cloth.

This practice cleans the inside lining of the stomach.

Definitely this practice should be learnt only from an expert teacher.

Frequency: Once a week on an empty stomach for general health. Daily if you suffer from asthma.

20

Surya Namaskara

This practice revitalizes the whole body and removes all signs of sleep, making it an excellent way to begin your yoga program. It loosens all the joints, flexes every muscle in the body and activates the respiratory and circulatory systems. It also balances the flow of prana in the ida and pingala nadis, providing optimum conditions for meditation. Its benefits are innumerable.

Surya namaskara consists of four essential aspects. All of them must be integrated in order to gain the best possible results from this practice.

1. *Physical postures*: There are twelve physical postures that correspond to the signs of the zodiac.
2. *Breathing*: Each position is associated either with inhalation, or retention or exhalation, so that the whole sequence is synchronized with breathing. This breath flow must not be forced or unnatural.
3. *Awareness*: This is as essential in surya namaskara as it is in all yogic practice. Without awareness most of the potential of this practice is lost.
4. *Relaxation*: Not strictly a part of surya namaskara itself, relaxation is necessary on completion of the practice to allow the body to return to normal. Shavasana with constant awareness of breath is the most recommended procedure.

Sequence for learning

One should first familiarize oneself with the twelve positions and for at least a week be concerned only with mastering the physical movements. Once you find that you can perform all the movements automatically, with little conscious direction, then synchronize the breath. Awareness should then be on both breath and movement. Finally, learn the mantras and try to synchronize them with each position.

One complete round

One full round consists of twenty-four positions. We have given twelve positions. These same twelve positions are to be repeated, but the opposite side of the body will now be treated, with the right leg lunging forward and the left leg extended backward in the relevant positions.

Tempo and number of rounds

At first surya namaskara should be performed slowly to ensure correct development of the movement and breathing. However, with regular practice your body will flow smoothly through the positions and you will be able to perform them faster. You may then speed up the practice but always ensure that the breath does not become shallow and that the mantras are correctly pronounced.

The number of rounds depends on individual health and time available. Surya namaskara should never be practised to exhaustion. Beginners should start with two rounds, adding one more round every second day. A person of reasonably good health should aim at twelve rounds a day, but the number of rounds is really a matter of individual capacity.

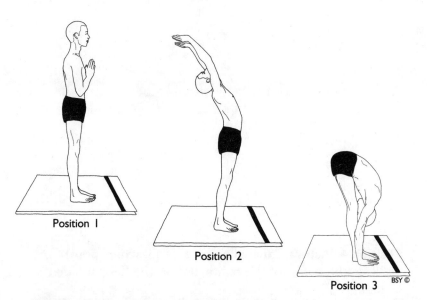

Position 1

Position 2

Position 3 BSY©

Position 1: Pranamasana (prayer pose)

Remain standing upright with the feet together.

Place the palms together in front of the chest in namaskara mudra.

Relax the whole body.

Breathing: Breathe normally.

Position 2: Hasta Utthanasana (raised arms pose)

Raise and stretch both arms above the head, separating the hands shoulder width apart.

Bend the head, arms and upper trunk backward slightly.

Breathing: Inhale while raising the arms.

Position 3: Padahastasana (hand to foot pose)

Bend forward until the fingers or palms of the hands touch the floor on either side of the feet.

Try to touch the knees with the forehead.

Do not strain.

Keep the knees straight.

Breathing: Exhale while bending forward.

Contra-indications: People with back conditions should not bend forward fully. Bend only as far as comfortable.

103

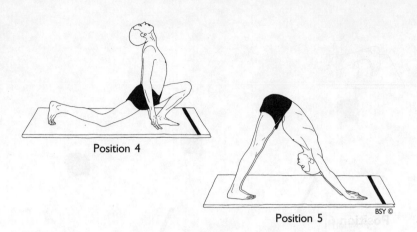

Position 4

Position 5

BSY ©

Position 4: Ashwa Sanchalanasana (equestrian pose)

Place the palms of the hands flat on the floor beside the feet.

Stretch the right leg back as far as possible.

At the same time, bend the left knee, keeping the left foot on the floor in the same position. Keep the arms straight. In the final position, the weight of the body should be supported on both hands, the left foot, right knee and toes of the right foot. The head should be tilted backward and the back arched.

Breathing: Inhale while stretching the right leg back.

Practice note: In the final pose the palms of the hands should be flat on the floor initially. Later on, more advanced practitioners may come up onto the fingertips.

Position 5: Parvatasana (mountain pose)

Take the left foot back beside the right foot.

Simultaneously, raise the buttocks and lower the head between the arms, so that the back and legs form two sides of a triangle.

The legs and arms should be straight in the final position.

Try to keep the heels on the floor in the final pose.

Do not strain.

Breathing: Exhale while taking the left leg back.

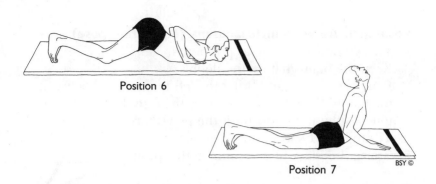

Position 6

Position 7

BSY ©

Position 6: Ashtanga Namaskara (salute with eight parts or points)

Lower the knees, chest and chin to the floor.

In the final position only the toes, knees, chest, hands and chin touch the floor. The knees, chest and chin should touch the floor simultaneously. If this is not possible, first lower the knees, then chest, and finally the chin. Buttocks, hips and abdomen should be raised.

Breathing: The breath is held outside in this pose. There is no respiration.

Position 7: Bhujangasana (cobra pose)

Lower the buttocks and hips to the floor.

Straightening the elbows, arch the back and push the chest forward into the cobra pose. Bend the head back. The thighs and hips remain on the floor and the arms support the trunk. Unless the spine is very flexible the arms will remain slightly bent.

Breathing: Inhale while raising the torso and arching the back.

Position 8: Parvatasana (mountain pose)

This stage is a repeat of position 5.

From bhujangasana assume parvatasana.

The hands and feet do not move from position 7.

Raise the buttocks and lower the heels to the floor.

Breathing: Exhale while raising the buttocks.

Position 9: Ashwa Sanchalanasana (equestrian pose)

This stage is the same as position 4.

Keep the palms flat on the floor.

Bend the left leg and bring the left foot forward between the hands. Simultaneously, lower the right knee so that it touches the floor and push the pelvis forward.

Tilt the head backward.

Breathing: Inhale while assuming the pose.

Position 10: Padahastasana (hand to foot pose)

This position is a repeat of position 3.

Bring the right foot forward next to the left foot.

Straighten both knees.

Bring the forehead as close to the knees as possible without straining.

Breathing: Exhale while performing the movement.

Position 11: Hasta Utthanasana (raised arms pose)

This stage is a repeat of position 2.

Raise the torso and stretch the arms above the head.

Keep the arms separated shoulder width apart.

Bend the head, arms and upper trunk backward slightly.

Breathing: Inhale while straightening the body.

Position 12: Pranamasana (prayer pose)

This is the final position and is the same as position 1.

Bring the palms together in front of the chest.

Breathing: Exhale while assuming the final position.

Positions 13–24: The twelve positions of surya namaskara are practised twice to complete one round. Positions 1 to 12 constitute half a round. In the second half, the positions are repeated with two small changes:
a) In position 16, instead of stretching the right foot backward, stretch the left foot back.
b) In position 21, bend the right leg and bring the right foot between the hands.

Conclusion: On the completion of each half round, lower the arms to the side, relax the body and concentrate on the breath until it returns to normal. After completing surya namaskara, practise shavasana for a few minutes.

Duration: Beginners should start with 2 or 3 rounds and add one more round every few weeks to a maximum of 12 rounds.

Contra-indications: The practice of surya namaskara should be immediately discontinued if a fever, acute inflammation, boils or rashes occur. These may develop due to excess toxins in the body. When the toxins have been eliminated, the practice may be resumed.

Surya namaskara should not be practised by people suffering from high blood pressure, coronary artery diseases, or those who have had a stroke. It should also be avoided in cases of hernia or intestinal tuberculosis.

People with back conditions should consult a medical expert before commencing this practice.

During the onset of menstruation, this practice should be avoided.

Note: For more information on this practice see the Bihar School of Yoga publication *Surya Namaskara: A Technique of Solar Revitalization*.

21

Pawanmuktasana Series

PART 1: ANTI RHEUMATIC GROUP

This series of exercises is especially designed for those people who have not practised yoga before and whose bodies are too stiff to attempt major asanas immediately on commencing yoga practice.

Physically speaking, these exercises are relatively undemanding. However, they must be practised as carefully as possible and with full awareness of movement and bodily sensation. Practised mindfully, they are very efficient and most powerful. They remove excessive wind and acid from the body.

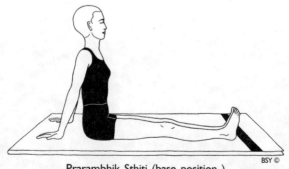

Prarambhik Sthiti (base position)

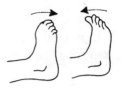

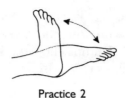

| Practice 1 | Practice 2 | Practice 3 |

Practice 1: Padanguli Naman (toe bending)

Sit in the base position ;with the legs outstretched and the feet slightly apart. Place the hands beside and slightly behind the buttocks.

Lean back a little, keep the spine straight, using the arms to support the back.

Move the toes of both feet slowly backward and forward, keeping the feet upright and the ankles relaxed and motionless. Hold each position for a few seconds.

Repeat 6–10 times.

Breathing: Inhale as the toes move backward. Exhale as the toes move forward.

Practice 2: Goolf Naman (ankle bending)

Remain in the base position. Keep the feet slightly apart. Slowly move both feet backward and forward, bending them from the ankle joints. Hold each position for a few seconds.

Repeat 6–10 times.

Breathing: Inhale as the feet move backward. Exhale as the feet move forward.

Practice 3: Goolf Chakra (ankle rotation)

Remain in the base position. Separate the legs a little, keeping them straight. Keep the heels on the ground throughout the practice.

Stage 1: Slowly rotate the right foot clockwise from the ankle 6–10 times and then repeat 6–10 times anti-clockwise.

Repeat the same procedure with the left foot.

109

Stage 2: Place the feet together. Slowly rotate both feet together in the same direction, keeping them in contact with each other. Do not allow the knees to move.

Practise 6–10 times clockwise and then 6–10 times anti-clockwise.

Breathing: Inhale on the upward movement. Exhale on the downward movement.

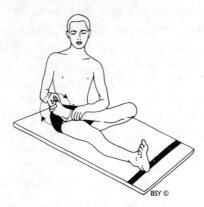

BSY ©

Practice 4: Goolf Ghoornan (ankle crank)

Remain in the base position.

Bend the right knee and place the foot on the left thigh with the ankle far enough over the thigh to be free for rotation. Hold the right ankle with the right hand.

Hold the toes of the right foot with the left hand.

With the left hand, slowly rotate the right foot 6–10 times clockwise, then 6–10 times anti-clockwise.

Repeat with the left foot placed on the right thigh.

Breathing: Inhale on the upward movement.

Exhale on the downward movement.

Practice 5: Janu Naman (knee bending)

Stay in the base position. Bend the right knee and clasp the hands under the right thigh.

Straighten the right leg, pulling up the kneecap.

Keep the hands under the thigh but straighten the arms. Do not allow the heel or toes to touch the floor.

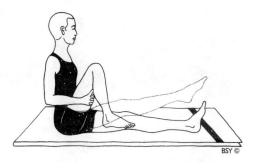

Bend the right leg at the knee so that the thigh comes close to the chest and the heel near the right buttock. This is one round.

Practise 6–10 rounds with the right leg and then 6–10 rounds with the left leg.

Breathing: Inhale while straightening the leg. Exhale while bending the leg.

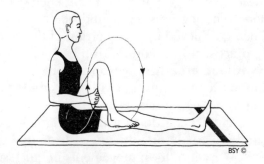

Practice 6: Janu Chakra (knee crank)

Sit in the base position.

Bend the right leg at the knee as described in practice 5. Place the hands under the right thigh and interlock the fingers or cross the arms holding the elbows.

Raise the right foot from the ground.

Rotate the lower leg from the knee in a large circular movement. The upper leg should be completely still.

Rotate 6–10 times clockwise and then 6–10 times anti-clockwise. Repeat with the left leg.

Breathing: Inhale on the upward movement.

Exhale on the downward movement.

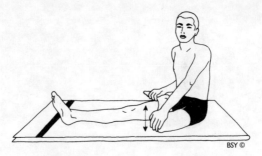

Practice 7: Ardha Titali Asana (half butterfly)

Sit in the base position. Bend the right leg and place the right foot as far up on the left thigh as possible.

Place the right hand on top of the bent right knee.

Hold the toes of the right foot with the left hand.

Stage 1: with breath synchronization

While inhaling, gently move the right knee up towards the chest. Exhaling, gently push the knee down towards the floor. The leg muscles should be passive, the movement being achieved by the exertion of the right arm.

Slowly practise 10 up and down movements.

Stage 2: without breath synchronization

Remain in the same position with the right leg on the left thigh and the leg muscles relaxed.

Push the right knee down with the right hand towards floor and release, letting the knee spring up by itself.

Practise 30 up and down movements in quick succession.

Breathing should be normal and unrelated to the practice.

Repeat stages 1 and 2 with the left leg.

Practice note: To unlock the leg after completing stage 2, bring the bent knee in front of the chest, then slowly and carefully straighten the leg.

Practice 8: Shroni Chakra (hip rotation)

Sit in the same starting position as for asana 7 with the right leg on the left thigh.

Using the muscles of the right arm, rotate the right knee in a large circle.

112

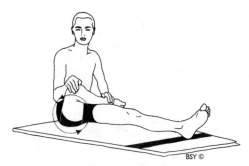

Practise 6–10 rotations clockwise and then 6–10 rotations anti-clockwise.

Release the knee as described in the practice note to asana 7.

Repeat with the left leg.

Breathing: Inhale on the upward movement.

Exhale on the downward movement.

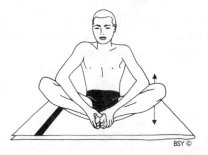

Practice 9: Poorna Titali Asana (full butterfly)

Sit in the base position.

Bend the knees and bring the soles of the feet together, keeping the heels as close to the body as possible.

Fully relax the inner thigh muscles.

Stage 1: Clasp the feet with both hands.

Gently bounce both knees up and down, pushing the knees towards the ground on the downward stroke.

If the legs are stiff use the elbows as levers to press the legs down.

Practise 30 to 50 up and down movements.

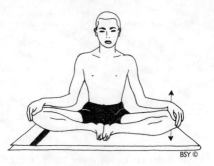

Stage 2: Keep the soles of the feet together.
Place the hands on the knees.
Using the palms, gently push the knees down towards the floor, then allowing them to spring up again.
Do not force this movement.
Repeat 20 to 30 times.
Straighten the legs and relax.
Breathing: Normal breathing, unrelated to the practice.
Contra-indications: People with sciatica and sacral conditions should avoid this asana.

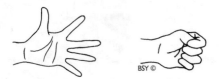

Practice 10: Mushtika Bandhana (hand clenching)
Sit in the base position or a cross-legged pose.
Hold both arms straight in front of the body at shoulder level. Open the hands, palms down, and stretch the fingers as wide apart as possible.
Slowly close the fingers with the thumbs inside to make a tight fist.
Again open the hands and stretch the fingers.
Repeat 6–10 times.
Breathing: Inhale on opening the hands. Exhale on closing the hands.

114

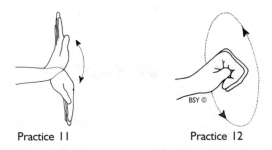

Practice 11   Practice 12

Practice 11: Manibandha Naman (wrist bending)

Remain in the base position or a cross-legged pose.

Stretch the arms in front of the body at shoulder level.

Keep the elbows straight, the palms open and fingers straight throughout the practice.

Bend the hands backward from the wrists as if pressing the palms against a wall with the fingers pointing toward the ceiling. Bend the hands forward from the wrists so that the fingers point toward the floor.

Bend the hands up again for the next round.

Repeat 6–10 times.

Breathing: Inhale with the backward movement. Exhale with the forward movement.

Practice 12: Manibandha Chakra (wrist joint rotation)

Remain in the base position or a comfortable cross-legged pose.

Stage 1: Extend the right arm forward at shoulder level.

Make a fist with the right hand, with the thumb inside.

Slowly rotate the fist about the wrist, ensuring that the palm faces downward throughout the rotation.

The arms and elbows should remain perfectly straight and still.

Practise 6–10 times clockwise and 6–10 times anti-clockwise. Repeat the same with the left fist.

Stage 2: Extend both arms in front of the body with the fists clenched. Rotate both fists together in the same direction.

Practise 6–10 times in each direction.

115

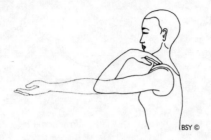

Practice 13: Kehuni Naman (elbow bending)

Stage 1: Remain sitting in the base position or a cross-legged pose. Stretch the arms in front of the body at shoulder level. The hands should be open with the palms facing up.

Bend the arms at the elbows and touch the fingers to the shoulders. Straighten the arms again. This is one round. Repeat 6–10 times.

Stage 2: Extend the arms sideways at shoulder level, hands open and palms up.

Bend the arms at the elbows and touch the fingers to the shoulders. Again straighten the arms sideways. Repeat 6–10 times.

Breathing: Inhale while straightening the arms. Exhale while bending the arms.

Practice note: The upper arms remain parallel to the floor, elbows at shoulder level.

Practice 14: Skandha Chakra (shoulder socket rotation)

Stage 1: Remain in the base position or a cross-legged pose.

Place the fingers of the right hand on the right shoulder. Rotate the right elbow in a large circle.

Practise 6–10 times lowering the elbow first and then 6–10 times raising the elbow.

Repeat with the left elbow.

Make sure that the head, trunk and spine remain straight and still.

116

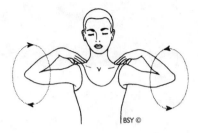

Stage 2: Place the fingers of the left hand on the left shoulder and the fingers of the right hand on the right shoulder. Fully rotate both elbows at the same time in a large circle.

Practise 6–10 times lowering the elbows first and then 6–10 times raising the elbows.

Breathing: Inhale on the upward stroke. Exhale on the downward stroke.

Practice 15: Greeva Sanchalana (neck movements)

Stage 1: Sit in the base position or a cross-legged pose with the hands resting on the knees. Close the eyes.

Slowly move the head forward and try to touch the chin to the chest. Then move the head as far back as comfortable. Do not strain.

Practise 3–7 times.

Breathing: Inhale on the backward movement. Exhale on the forward movement.

Stage 2: Remain in the same position, keeping the eyes closed.

Face directly forward.

Slowly move the head to the right bringing the right ear towards the right shoulder without turning the head or raising the shoulders.

Move the head to the left side bringing the left ear towards the left shoulder.

This is one round. Practise 3–7 rounds.

Breathing: Inhale on the upward movement. Exhale on the downward movement.

117

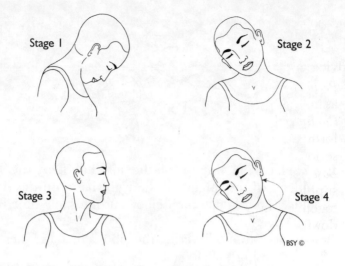

Stage 1

Stage 2

Stage 3

Stage 4

BSY ©

Stage 3: Remain in the base position.

Keep the head upright and the eyes closed.

Gently turn the head to the right so that the chin stays in line with the shoulder. Slowly turn the head to the left as far as is comfortable. Keep the chin at the same level from the floor throughout. Do not strain.

Practise 3–7 times on each side.

Breathing: Inhale while turning to the front. Exhale while turning to the side.

Stage 4: Remain in the same position with the eyes closed.

Slowly rotate the head, first downward, then to the right, backward and then to the left side in a relaxed, smooth, rhythmic, circular movement.

Practise 3–5 times clockwise and then 3–5 times anti-clockwise.

Do not strain.

After the practice, keep the neck straight and the eyes closed.

Breathing: Inhale as the head moves up. Exhale as the head moves down.

Contra-indications: Stage 4 should not be performed by elderly people and those suffering from low blood pressure, very high blood pressure or cervical spondylosis.

118

PART 2: DIGESTIVE/ABDOMINAL GROUP

Advice and precautions

- *Periodic rest*: A short rest should be taken between each asana, lying in shavasana.
- *Contra-indications*: These practices should not be performed by people suffering from high blood pressure, serious heart conditions, sciatica or slipped disc.
- *Base position*: All these asanas are performed from the supine position, lying flat on the back with the legs together and straight and the arms by the sides, palms down.

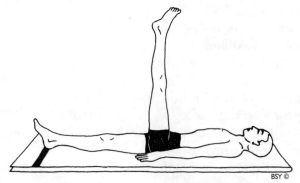

Practice 1: Utthanpadasana (raised legs pose)

Lie in the base position with the palms flat on the floor.
Inhale and raise the right leg as high as is comfortable, keeping it straight and the foot relaxed.
The left leg should remain straight and in contact with the floor.
Hold the posture for 3 to 5 seconds, retaining the breath.
Exhale and slowly lower the leg to the floor.
This is one round. Practise 5 rounds with the right leg and then 5 rounds with the left leg.
This may be repeated raising both legs together.

Breathing: Inhale while raising the leg(s).
Hold the posture and the breath. Exhale while lowering the leg(s).

119

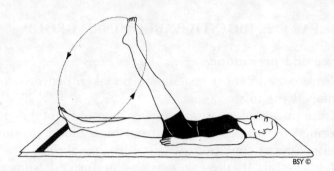

Practice 2: Chakra Padasana (leg rotation)

Lie in the base position.

Raise the right leg 5 cm from the ground, keeping the knee straight.

Rotate the entire leg clockwise 3–8 times in as large a circle as possible.

The heel should not touch the floor at any time during the rotation.

Rotate 3–8 times in the opposite direction.

Repeat with the left leg.

Do not strain. Rest in the base position until the respiration returns to normal.

Breathing: Breathe normally throughout the practice.

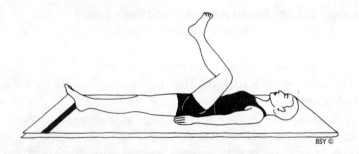

Practice 3: Pada Sanchalanasana (cycling)

Stage 1: Lie in the base position.

Bend the right knee and bring the thigh to the chest.

Raise and straighten the leg completely.

Then, lower the straight leg in a forward movement.

120

Bend the knee and bring it back to the chest to complete the cycling movement.

The heel should not touch the floor during the movement.

Repeat 3–8 times in a forward direction and then 3–8 times in reverse.

Repeat with the left leg.

Breathing: Inhale while bending the knee and bringing the thigh to the chest.

Exhale while lowering the leg.

Stage 2: Raise both legs.

Practise alternate cycling movements as though peddling a bicycle.

Practise 3–8 times in the forward direction and then 3–8 times backward.

Breathing: Breathe normally throughout.

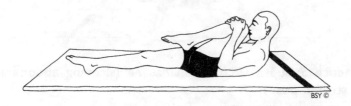

Practice 4: Supta Pawanmuktasana (leg lock pose)

Stage 1: Lie in the base position.

Bend the right knee and bring the thigh to the chest.

Interlock the fingers and clasp the hands on the shin just below the right knee.

Keep the left leg straight and on the ground.

Inhale deeply, then while exhaling raise the head and shoulders off the ground and try to touch the right knee with the nose. Hold the breath out in the final position for a few seconds, counting mentally.

While slowly inhaling, return to the base position.

Relax the body.

Repeat 3 times with the right leg and then 3 times with the left leg.

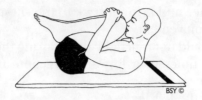

Stage 2: Remain in the base position.

Bend both knees and bring the thighs to the chest.
Interlock the fingers and clasp the hands on the shinbones just below the knees.
Practise the same movement as in stage 1 but with both legs together.
Practise this 3 times.

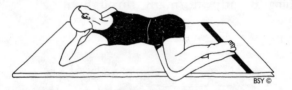

Practice 5: Supta Udarakarshanasana (sleeping abdominal stretch pose)

Lie in the base pose.
Bend the knees and place the soles of both feet flat on the ground, directly in front of the buttocks.
Keep the knees and feet together and the shoulders and elbows on the floor throughout the practice.
Interlock the fingers of both hands and place the palms under the back of the head. Inhale.
While breathing out, slowly lower the legs to the right, trying to bring the knees down to the floor. At the same time, gently turn the head and neck in the opposite direction to the legs.
Hold the breath out in the final position while mentally counting three seconds.
While breathing in, raise both legs and bring the head to the upright position.

Repeat on the left side to complete one round.

Practise 5 complete rounds.

Variation: Practise the same movement but start with the thighs up on the chest, feet off the floor.

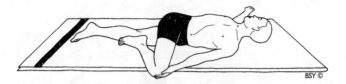

Practice 6: Shava Udarakarshanasana (universal spinal twist)

Lie down flat on the back and bring the legs and feet together.

Stretch the arms out to the sides at shoulder level with the palms facing down.

Bend the right leg and place the sole of the foot beside the left kneecap.

Place the left hand on top of the right knee.

This is the starting position.

Gently bring the right knee down to the floor on the left side of the body, keeping the leg bent and the foot in contact with the left knee.

The left leg should remain straight.

Turn the head to the right, look along the arm at the right hand.

The right arm and shoulder should remain in contact with the floor.

Hold the position for as long as is comfortable.

Return to the starting position, bringing the head and knee to the centre.

Stretch the right arm out to the side and straighten the right leg.

Repeat on the opposite side.

Practise once to each side, gradually extending the holding time.

123

Breathing: Inhale in the starting position.

Exhale while pushing the knee to the floor and turning the head.

Breathe deeply and slowly in the final position.

Inhale while centring the body and exhale while straightening the leg.

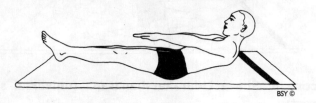

BSY ©

Practice 7: Naukasana (boat pose)

Lie in the base position, palms down. Keep the eyes open throughout.

Breathe in deeply. Hold the breath and then raise the legs, arms, shoulders, head and trunk off the ground.

The shoulders and feet should be no more than 15 cm off the floor.

The arms should be held at the same level and in line with the toes.

Remain in the final position and hold the breath.

Breathe out and return to the supine position. Relax the whole body.

This is one round.

Practise 3 to 5 rounds.

Relax in shavasana after each round.

Variation: Repeat the same process as above but tense the whole body in the raised position.

Contra-indications: Not be performed by persons with high blood pressure.

PART 3: SHAKTI BANDHA ASANAS

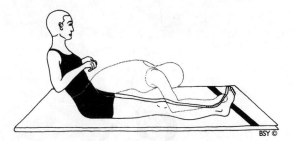

Nauka Sanchalanasana (rowing the boat)

Sit with both legs straight in front of the body.

Imagine the action of rowing a boat.

Clench the hands as though grasping oars, with the palms facing down.

Breathing out, straighten and raise the arms and bend forward from the waist as far as is comfortable. The legs should be kept straight.

Breathing in, lean back as far as possible, drawing the hands back towards the shoulders.

This is one round.

The hands should make a complete circular movement in every round, moving up the sides of the legs and trunk.

Practise 5 to 10 rounds.

Reverse the direction of the rowing movement.

Practise 5 to 10 times.

Breathing: Inhale while leaning back.
Exhale while bending forward.

Kashtha Takshanasana (chopping wood)

Sit in the squatting position with the feet flat on the floor one and a half feet apart and the knees separated.

Clasp the fingers of both hands together and place them on the floor between the feet with the elbows inside the knees.

Keep the arms straight throughout the practice.

125

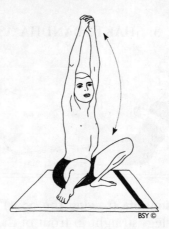

Raise the arms as high as possible above and behind the head, stretching the spine upward. Look up towards the hands.

Make a downward stroke with the arms, as if chopping wood. Expel the breath making a 'Ha!' sound to remove all the air from the lungs. The hands should return to the floor in between the feet and the head is facing forward.

This is one round.

Practise 5 to 10 rounds.

Breathing: Inhale while raising the arms.

Exhale while lowering the arms.

Practice note: This practice can also be done in the standing position.

Udarakarshanasana (abdominal stretch pose)

Sit in the squatting position with the feet apart and the hands on the knees.

Breathe in deeply.

Breathe out, bringing the right knee to the floor near the left foot.

Using the left hand as a lever, push the left knee towards the right side, simultaneously twisting to the left.

Try to squeeze the lower abdomen with the combined pressure of both thighs.

126

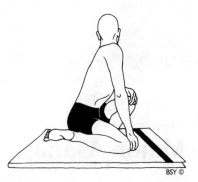

Look over the left shoulder.
Hold the breath out for 3 to 5 seconds in the final position.
Breathe in when returning to the starting position.
Repeat on the other side of the body to complete one round.
Practise 5 rounds.

Variation: Those who have difficulty balancing may support their backs against a wall while squatting. The heels should be about 20 cm from the wall to allow for the twist.

Practice note: This is one of the asanas performed in shankhaprakshalana.

22

Major Asanas

The meaning of the Sanskrit word *asana* is a steady or comfortable posture, not simply physical exercises. Asanas have a profound influence on the mind and consciousness as well as the body, moulding all three into a harmonious whole. One should, therefore, see asanas not as mere physical poses but as states of being, for their correct performance requires participation of one's whole being. One should be aware of oneself in relation to the physical position and movement, the breath, relaxation of the muscles and so on.

The aim of asana practice is to help us tread the path to higher awareness by eliminating bodily disease and imbalances. By promoting physical health, asanas also bring about mental changes, giving rise to calmness and optimism.

Asanas loosen the joints of the body, stretch and tone the muscles, remove toxins which tend to accumulate in various parts of the system, harmonize the nervous system and massage the internal organs to promote improved functioning. These practices tone the glands and balance the various hormones. They co-ordinate all metabolic complexes including the respiratory, digestive and circulatory systems. All these systems are rhythmical in nature and intimately connected with each other. Asanas regulate all these systems, bringing rhythm and harmony to both body and mind. The pranic or subtle body that energizes the physical body is also influenced by asanas, which encourage the free flow of vital energy, giving bodily vigor and mental equilibrium.

Advice and precautions
Place of practice: The place of practice should be clean, quiet and well ventilated. There should be no bad smell or dampness. The area should be cleared of furniture and other objects. A blanket or rug should be placed on the floor. Neither use a spongy mattress nor practise on the bare floor. Try to use the same place every day to build up an atmosphere of peace.

Clothing: Clothing should be as light as possible so free movement is not impeded. Before commencing your practices, remove your spectacles, wristwatch and any ornaments or jewellery.

Time of practice: The bowels and bladder should preferably be empty during the practice and the stomach must definitely be empty. To ensure this, allow three to four hours after eating food. It is thus best to practise in the early morning before breakfast. This also allows the practitioner to take advantage of brahmamuhurta (between four and six a.m.), which is the time of day most conducive to yoga practices. Although the body is stiffer early in the morning, there are fewer distractions and the atmosphere is pure and quiet. However, asanas can be practised at any time of the day except after meals.

Duration: Length of practice should be regulated according to the available time. Don't set your aims too high in the beginning; only do as much practice as you can do regularly, every day, without fail. Fifteen minutes practice every day is better than one hour of practice one day, then none for three days and again one hour.

Sequence: You should begin your program with asanas followed by pranayama and then meditation. Of course, if time is limited, you can begin meditation without preliminary practices.

129

Limitations: Don't practise asanas if you are ill with a cold, diarrhoea or something similar. At these times the body is directing its energy to specific areas to fight the illness; let it perform its duties unimpeded.

Slow, controlled movements: In order to bring harmony and to gain the most benefit from asanas they should be practised with slow, controlled movements that are co-ordinated with the breath. Fast movements imply excessive tension, and quick, sudden movements use up excessive energy. Asanas aim at conserving energy and developing muscular control, both of which come from slow, mindful practice. During slow movements, it is possible to relax the maximum number of muscles that are not directly involved in the particular asana. Breathing instructions have been included to facilitate this coordination and relaxation, and they should be followed as closely as possible. Breathe only through the nose.

Maintenance of final position: The final position is the most important part of the practice. This period of immobility is the time when profound and beneficial changes are occurring in the body.

Relaxation: Never exert undue force or strain while doing asanas. Though most beginners will find their muscles stiff to start with, they will definitely become more supple with regular practice. In order to stretch the muscles it is important to relax them as much as possible. If your muscles are tense, they will automatically resist any attempt to stretch them.

Relaxation between asanas is just as important as the asana itself. When one completely relaxes the organs and muscles return to their normal shape and they are flooded with purified blood to replace that squeezed out during performance of the asana. During this rest period the circulatory and respiratory systems also return to normal.

All asanas are postures for relaxation. However, shavasana is a highly recommended resting pose and should be practised between asanas. It is also an important part of

130

many short relaxation techniques, giving balanced support to the spine.

Awareness: While learning the asana your attention should be on correct performance. In the final position you can be aware of the breath, chakra or particular parts of the body that the asana especially influences. Such awareness is most useful in directing the body's natural healing energies. Asanas are a powerful force in healing. They work on many different levels, although you must experience this for yourself. It is only through experience that you come to understand the relief from suffering that comes with the regular practice of yogic poses. Under the guidance of a competent teacher, diseases such as asthma and diabetes can become problems of the past.

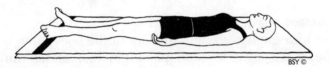

Shavasana (corpse pose)

Lie flat on the back with the arms about 15 cm away from the body, palms facing upward. A thin pillow or folded cloth may be placed behind the head to prevent discomfort. Let the fingers curl up slightly.

Move the feet slightly apart to a comfortable position and close the eyes.

The head and spine should be in a straight line.

Make sure the head does not fall to one side or the other.

Relax the whole body and stop all physical movement.

Become aware of the natural breath and allow it to become rhythmic and relaxed.

Duration: According to time available. In general, the longer the better although a minute or two is sufficient between asana practices.

Practice note: Try not to move the body at all during the practice.

131

MEDITATION ASANAS

In all the meditation asanas, either the left or the right leg
may be placed uppermost. Ideally, the leg position should
be alternated. A small cushion may be placed under the
buttocks.

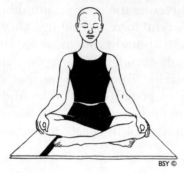

Sukhasana (easy pose)

Sit with the legs straight in front of the body.
Bend the right leg and place the foot under the left
thigh. Bend the left leg and place the foot under the
right thigh.
Place the hands on the knees with the arms relaxed
Make the head, neck and back upright and straight.
Close the eyes and relax the whole body.
Variation: Sukhasana may also be performed sitting cross-
legged with a belt or cloth tied around the knees and
lower back.

Siddhasana (accomplished pose for men)

Sit with the legs straight in front of the body.
Bend the right leg and place the sole of the foot flat
against the inner left thigh with the heel pressing the
perineum, the area midway between the genitals and the
anus.
Bend the left leg and place the left ankle directly over the
right ankle so that the anklebones are touching and
the heels are one above the other.

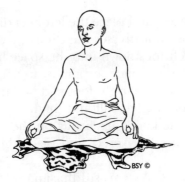

Press the pubis with the left heel directly above the
genitals.
Push the toes and the outer edge of the left foot into the
space between the right calf and thigh muscles.
Grasp the toes of the right foot and pull them up into the
space between the left calf and thigh.
The legs should now be locked with the knees touching
the ground.
Make the spine erect and place the hands on the knees.

Contra-indications: Siddhasana should not be practised
by those with sciatica or sacral infections.

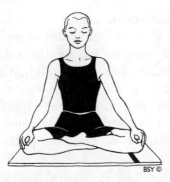

Siddha Yoni Asana (accomplished pose for women)
Sit with the legs straight in front of the body.
Bend the right leg and place the sole of the foot flat
against the inner left thigh. Place this heel firmly against
or inside the labia majora of the vagina.

Bend the left leg and place the left heel directly on top of the right heel so it presses the clitoris.

Wedge the left toes down into the space between the calf and thigh so they touch, or almost touch, the floor.

Grasp the toes of the right foot and pull them up into the space between the left calf and thigh.

Ensure that the knees are firmly on the ground.

Make the spine fully erect and place the hands on the knees.

Contra-indications: As for siddhasana.

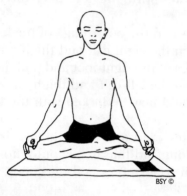

Swastikasana (auspicious pose)

Sit with the legs straight in front of the body.

Bend the left knee and place the sole of the left foot against the inside of the right thigh. There is no contact between the heel and the perineum.

Bend the right knee and place the right foot in the space between the left thigh and calf muscle. There is no contact between the heel and the pubis.

Grasp the toes of the left foot and pull them up into the space between the right calf and thigh.

The knees should be firmly on the floor.

Straighten the spine and place the hands on top of the knees.

Variation: After bending the left leg and placing the sole against the inside of the right thigh, bend the right leg and place the heel of the right foot on the floor in front of the left foot with the sole resting against the left shin. Place the hands on the knees.

Contra-indications: Swastikasana should not be performed by people with sciatica or sacral infections.

VAJRASANA GROUP OF ASANAS

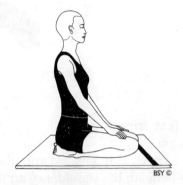

Vajrasana (thunderbolt pose)

Kneel on the floor.

Bring the big toes together and separate the heels.

Lower the buttocks onto the inside surface of the feet with the heels touching the sides of the hips.

Place the hands on the knees, palms down.

The back and head should be straight

Breathe normally and fix the attention on the flow of air at the nostrils.

Duration: Practise vajrasana as much as possible, especially directly after meals, for at least 5 minutes, to enhance the digestive function.

Practice note: A folded blanket or small cushion may be placed between the buttocks and the heel.

Variation: Place a rolled up blanket on the floor between the legs. Separate the feet (not the knees) about 25cm. Sit on the blanket in vajrasana.

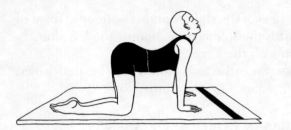

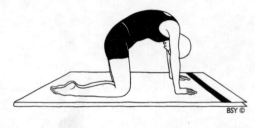

Marjari-asana (cat stretch pose)

Sit in vajrasana.

Stand on the knees, lean forward and place the hands flat on the floor beneath the shoulders with the fingers facing forward.

The hands should be in line with the knees; the arms and thighs should be perpendicular to the floor.

Inhale while raising the head and depressing the spine so that the back becomes concave.

Exhale, while lowering the head and stretching the spine upward.

At the end of exhalation pull in the buttocks.

The head will now be between the arms, facing the thighs.

This is one round.

Breathing: Try to perform the movement breathing as slowly as possible.

Duration: Perform 5 to 10 full rounds for general purposes.

Practice note: Do not bend the arms at the elbows. Keep the arms and thighs vertical throughout.

136

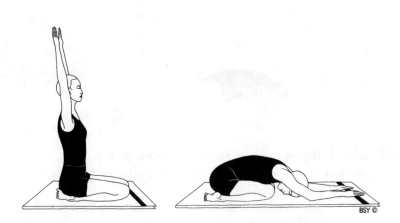

Shashankasana (pose of the moon or hare pose)

Sit in vajrasana, placing the palms on the thighs just above the knees.

While inhaling, raise the arms above the head, keeping them straight and shoulder width apart.

Exhale while bending the trunk forward from the hips, keeping the arms and head in line with the trunk.

At the end of the movement, the hands and forehead should rest on the floor in front of the knees.

If possible, the arms and forehead should touch the floor at the same time.

Bend the arms slightly and let the elbows rest on the floor. Retain the breath out for up to 5 seconds in the final position. Then, simultaneously inhale and slowly raise the arms and trunk to the vertical position.

Breathe out while lowering the arms to the knees.

This is one round.

Practise 3 to 5 rounds.

Duration: Beginners should slowly increase the length of time in the final position after the last round until they are able to hold it comfortably for 3–10 minutes, breathing normally.

Contra-indications: Not to be performed by people with very high blood pressure, slipped disc or those who suffer from vertigo.

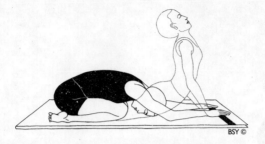

Shashank Bhujangasana (striking cobra pose)

Assume marjari-asana, placing the palms flat on the floor beneath the shoulders.

Move into shashankasana with the arms outstretched in front of the shoulders.

Then, slowly move the chest forward sliding it just above the floor until it is in line with the hands.

Move the chest further forward and then upward, straightening the arms, at the same time lowering the pelvis to the floor.

In the final position, the arms should be straight, the back arched and the head raised as in bhujangasana.

Hold this position for a few seconds, retaining the breath.

Slowly raise the buttocks and move backwards, keeping the arms straight, return to shashankasana.

This is one round. Relax the whole body for a short time before starting another round.

Practise 5 to 7 rounds.

Breathing: Inhale on the forward movement.

Hold the breath for a few seconds in the final position.

Exhale while returning to shashankasana.

Practice note: The hand position should not change during the entire practice.

Pranamasana (bowing pose)

Sit in vajrasana. Grasp the lower calves just above the ankles, keeping the thumbs uppermost.

Slowly bend forward and place the crown of the head on the floor in front of the knees. (Place a small folded blanket under the head).

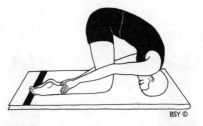

Raise the buttocks as high as possible, until the thighs are as vertical as possible.

Remain in the final position for 5 to 20 seconds.

Lower the buttocks and come back into shashankasana for a short time before returning to vajrasana.

Practise this asana 5 times.

Breathing: Inhale in the position of vajrasana and while raising the buttocks.

Exhale while lowering the head to the floor.

Hold the breath in the final position or breathe normally if remaining in the position for more than a few seconds.

Contra-indications: This asana should not be performed by those who suffer from vertigo, weak neck or high blood pressure.

STANDING ASANAS

Hasta Utthanasana (hand raising pose)

Stand erect with the feet together and the arms by the sides.

Cross the hands in front of the body.

Inhale deeply and slowly raise the arms above the head, keeping the hands crossed.

Synchronise the movement with the breath.

At the same time, bend the head slightly backward and look up at the hands.

Exhale and spread the arms out to the sides so that they form a straight line at shoulder level.

Inhale and reverse the movement, re-crossing the arms above the head.

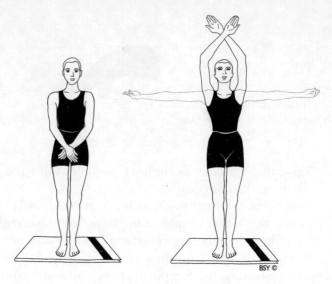

Exhale and lower the arms straight down the front of the body so that they are once again in the starting position. Repeat the process 5 to 10 times.

Tadasana (palm tree pose)

Stand with the feet together or about 10 cm apart, and the arms by the sides.

Raise the arms over the head, interlock the fingers, turning the palms upward, and place the hands on top of the head.

Keep the eyes fixed on a point on the wall slightly above head level.

Inhale and stretch the arms, shoulders and chest upward.

Raise the heels coming up onto the toes. Stretch the whole body, holding the breath and the position for a few seconds.

Lower the heels while breathing out and bring the hands back to the top of the head.

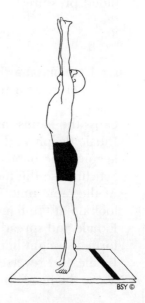

This is one round.

Practise 5 to 10 rounds.

Breathing: The breath should be synchronised with the raising and lowering of the arms.

Variation: Tadasana may also be performed while gazing up at the interlocked fingers.

Note : *This is one of the asanas for shankhaprakshalana.*

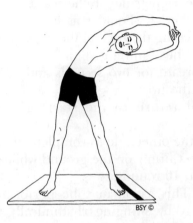

Tiryaka Tadasana (swaying palm tree pose)

Stand with the feet about 2 feet apart. Fix the gaze on a point in front. Interlock the fingers and turn the palms outward. Inhale and raise the arms over the head.

While exhaling, bend to the left side from the waist.

Do not bend forward or backward or twist the trunk.

Hold the position for a few seconds while retaining the breath outside. Inhale and slowly come to the upright position. Repeat on the right side.

From the upright position exhale while bringing the arms down to the sides. This completes one round.

Practise 5 to 10 rounds.

Variation: The fingers may be interlocked with the palms facing downward.

Note : *This is one of the asanas for shankhaprakshalana.*

141

Kati Chakrasana (waist rotating pose)

Stand with the feet about half a metre apart and the arms by the sides.

Take a deep breath in while raising the arms to shoulder level. Breathe out and twist the body to the left.

Bring the right hand to the left shoulder and wrap the left arm around the back to the right side of the waist. Look over the left shoulder as far as possible, keeping the back of the neck straight and head upright.

Hold the breath for two seconds and accentuate the twist.

Inhale and return to the starting position.

Repeat on the other side to complete one round.

Keep the feet firmly on the ground while twisting.

Practise 5 to 10 rounds.

Practice note: This asana may be performed in a more dynamic way by swinging rhythmically with the arms without synchronizing the movements with the breath.

Note: *This is one of the asanas for shankhaprakshalana.*

Dwikonasana (double angle pose)

Stand erect with the feet one foot apart.

Extend the arms behind the back and interlock the fingers.

Bend forward from the hips while simultaneously raising the arms behind the back as high as possible without strain. Keep the arms straight.

Look forward as far as possible, so that the face is parallel with the floor.

Remain in the final position for a short time and return to the upright position.

Relax the arms.

Repeat up to 5 times.

142

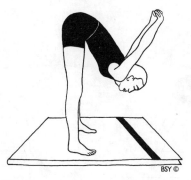

Breathing: Inhale while standing erect and when returning to the upright position.

Exhale while bending forward.

Contra-indications: In acute or painful conditions of the shoulder joints this asana should be avoided.

Trikonasana (triangle pose)

Variation 1: Stand erect with the feet about a metre apart. Turn the right foot to the right side.

Stretch the arms sideways and raise them to shoulder level so that they are in one straight line.

Bend to the right. Simultaneously bend the right knee slightly.

Place the right hand on the right foot, keeping the two arms in line with each other.

Look up at the left hand in the final position.

Return to the upright position with the arms in a straight line. Repeat on the opposite side.

This completes one round.

Practise 5 rounds.

Variation 2: Repeat the basic form, but instead of keeping the upper arm vertical in the final position, lower it over the ear until it is parallel to the floor with the palm facing down.

Repeat on the left side.

Breathing: Inhale while raising the arms. Exhale while bending.

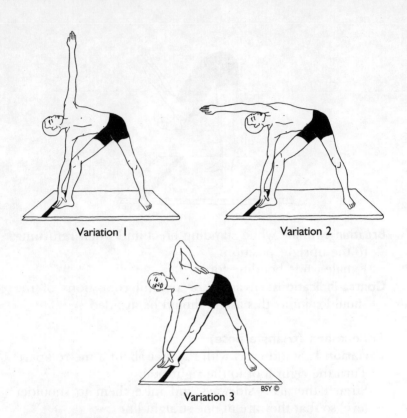

Variation 1

Variation 2

Variation 3

BSY ©

Hold the breath for a few seconds in the final position.
Inhale while raising the body to the vertical position.

Variation 3: Stand with the feet one metre apart and the toes facing forward.

Place the palms of the hands on each side of the waist with the fingers pointing downward.

Breathing out, slowly bend to the right from the hips while sliding the right hand down along the outside of the right thigh as far as is comfortable. Keep the legs straight.

Stay in the final position for a few seconds, holding the breath out.

Raise the trunk to the upright position while breathing in, and return the right hand to the waist.

Repeat on the left side to complete one round.

Practise 3 to 5 rounds.

144

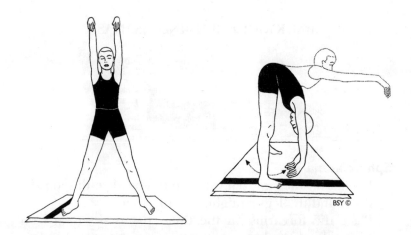

Utthita Lolasana (swinging while standing pose)

Stand erect with the feet a metre apart.

Raise the arms over the head keeping the elbows straight.
Bend the wrists forward so that the hands hang limp.

Bend forward and swing the trunk down from the hips,
allowing the arms and head to swing through the legs.

Be tension-free like a rag doll. On the upward swing,
raise the trunk so that it is parallel to the floor.

On the downward swing bring the hands as far back as
possible behind the feet.

After 5 complete swings return to the upright position
with the arms raised, then lower the arms to the sides.

Repeat up to 5 times.

Breathing: Inhale fully through the nose while raising the
arms and while returning to the upright position.

Exhale forcefully through the mouth on each downward
swing to expel all the air from the lower lungs.

For added effect, the sound 'ha' may be made with each
forced exhalation. This sound should come from the
abdomen.

Contra-indications: This asana is not to be practised by
people who suffer from vertigo, high blood pressure or
back conditions.

BACKWARD BENDING ASANAS

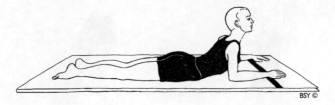

Sphinx asana

Lie flat on the stomach with the forehead resting on the floor, and the legs straight, feet together.

Place the forearms on the floor, palms downward on each side of the head. The fingers point forward in line with the crown of the head. The forearms and elbows are close to the body.

Raise the head, shoulders and chest by bringing the upper arms to the vertical position.

The elbows, forearms and hands remain on the floor.

Relax in the position for a comfortable length of time and then slowly lower the body.

This is one round.

Breathing: Inhale while raising the head, shoulders and chest.

Exhale while lowering to the floor.

Breathe normally in the final position.

Duration: Hold the position for 3 to 4 minutes as a static pose or practise up to 5 rounds as a dynamic pose.

Bhujangasana (cobra pose)

Lie flat on the stomach with the legs straight and feet together, and the forehead on the floor.

Place the palms of the hands flat on the floor under the shoulders.

Slowly raise the head, neck and shoulders, then using the back muscles start to raise the trunk.

Then begin using the arm muscles and raise the trunk further, straightening the elbows to raise the trunk as

146

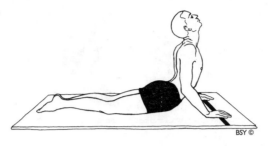

high as possible and arch the back. Gently tilt the head backward.

In the final position, the pubic bone remains in contact with the floor. The arms may or may not be straight depending on flexibility.

Hold the final position.

To return to the starting position, slowly bring the head forward, release the upper back by bending the arms and lower the navel, chest, shoulders and finally the forehead to the floor.

This is one round.

Breathing: Inhale while raising the torso.

Breathe normally in the final position or retain the breath if the pose is held for a short time.

Exhale while lowering the torso.

Duration: Practise up to 5 rounds, gradually increasing the length of time in the final position.

Contra-indications: People suffering from peptic ulcer, hernia, intestinal tuberculosis or hyperthyroidism should not practise this asana without expert guidance.

Tiryaka Bhujangasana (twisting cobra pose)

Assume the final position of bhujangasana with the legs separated about half a metre; the toes should also be tucked under and the heels raised.

The head should be facing forward not bending backward.

Twist the head and upper portion of the trunk, and look over the left shoulder at the heel of the right foot.

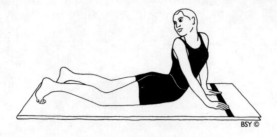

Stay in the final position for a few seconds.

Face forward again and repeat the twist on the other side without lowering the trunk.

Return to the centre and lower the body to the floor.

This is one round.

Breathing: Inhale while raising.

Retain the breath inside while twisting to both sides.

Exhale while lowering to the floor.

Duration: Practise 3 to 5 rounds.

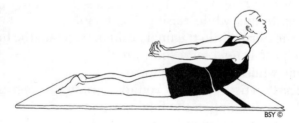

Sarpasana (snake pose)

Lie flat on the stomach with the legs straight and the feet together.

Interlock the fingers and place the hands on top of the buttocks. Place the chin on the floor.

This is the starting position.

Using the lower back muscles, raise the chest as far as possible from the floor. Push the hands back and raise the arms as high as possible. Squeeze the shoulder blades together.

Hold for as long as is comfortable.

148

Slowly return to the starting position and relax the whole body. Release the hands and relax the arms by the sides of the body. Turn the head to one side.

This is one round.

Breathing: Inhale deeply and slowly in the starting position prior to raising.

Retain while raising and in the final position.

Exhale while lowering.

Duration: Up to 5 rounds.

Contra-indications: People with heart conditions and high blood pressure should take care not to strain while performing this asana.

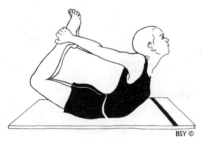

BSY ©

Dhanurasana (bow pose)

Lie flat on the stomach with the legs and feet together, and the arms and hands beside the body.

Bend the knees and bring the heels close to the buttocks. Clasp the hands around the ankles. Place the chin on the floor. This is the starting position.

Using the leg muscles and keeping the arms straight, push the feet away from the body. Arch the neck and back, lifting the thighs, chest and head together.

Hold the final position for as long as is comfortable and then, slowly lower the legs, chest and head to the starting position.

Release the starting position and relax until the respiration returns to normal.

This is one round.

Breathing: Inhale deeply in the starting position.
Retain the breath while raising the body.
Retain the breath inside in the final position.
Exhale while returning to the prone position.
Duration: 3 to 5 rounds.
Contra-indications: People who suffer from a weak heart, high blood pressure, hernia, colitis, peptic or duodenal ulcers should not attempt this practice.

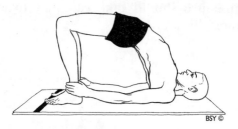

Kandharasana (shoulder pose)

Lie flat on the back. Bend the knees, placing the soles of the feet flat on the floor with the heels touching the buttocks. Grasp the ankles with the hands.
This is the starting position.
Raise the buttocks and arch the back upward.
Try to raise the chest and navel as high as possible, pushing the chest up towards the chin and head without moving the position of the feet or shoulders.
Hold the pose for as long as is comfortable and then lower the body to the starting position.
Release the ankles and relax with the legs outstretched.
Breathing: Inhale deeply in the starting position.
Retain the breath inside while raising and holding the final position.
Alternatively, breathe slowly and deeply in the final position.
Exhale while lowering to the starting position.
Duration: Practise 5 to 10 rounds.

Contra-indications: People suffering from peptic or duodenal ulcers, or abdominal hernia should not practise this asana.

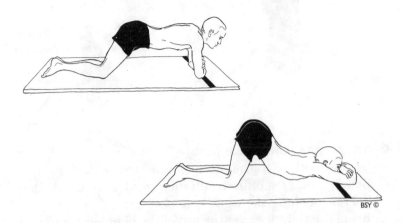

Utthan Pristhasana (lizard pose)

Lie on the stomach with the arms crossed under the chest, each hand holding the opposite upper arm. The elbows should not move during the practice.

Separate the legs slightly.

The head faces forward.

This is the starting position.

Raise the trunk and buttocks so that the body is supported by the knees and elbows.

Stretch the torso back, placing the chin and chest on, or as close as possible to, the floor behind the forearms.

Return to the raised position and then back to the starting position.

This is one round.

Breathing: Inhale while raising the buttocks (twice during each round). Exhale while lowering the buttocks (twice during each round).

Duration: Up to 10 rounds, or hold the final position with the chest on the floor for 10 breaths.

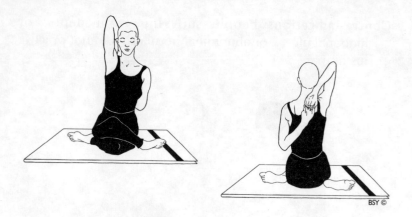

Gomukhasana (cow's face pose)

Sit with both legs straight in front of the body.

Bend the left leg underneath the right leg so that the left heel is touching the right buttock.

Bring the right leg over the top of the bent left leg so that the right heel touches the left buttock.

Adjust the right knee so that it is above the left knee.

Place the left arm behind the back and the right arm over the right shoulder.

Try to clasp the fingers of both hands behind the back.

Bring the raised elbow behind the head so that the head presses against the inside of the raised arm.

The spine should be erect and the head back. Close the eyes.

Stay in this position for up to 2 minutes.

Unclasp the hands, straighten the legs and repeat with the left knee uppermost and the left arm over the left shoulder.

Breathing: Normal in the final position.

Matsyasana (fish pose)

Sit in padmasana and relax the whole body.

Carefully bend backward, supporting the body with the arms and elbows. Lift the chest slightly, take the head back and lower the crown of the head to the floor.

152

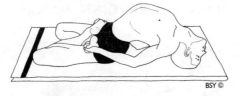

Hold the big toes and rest the elbows on the floor.
Allow the head, buttocks and legs to support the weight of the body.
Return to the starting position, reversing the order of movements.
Repeat the asana, with the legs crossed the other way.

Duration: The final position may be held up to 1 to 3 minutes.

Breathing: Breathe deeply and slowly in the final position.

Contra-indications: People who suffer from heart disease, peptic ulcers, hernia, back conditions or any serious illness should not practise this asana.

Practice note: It is important that the body is slowly lowered into and raised from the final position by using the arms.

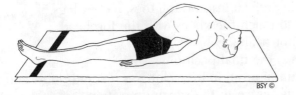

Variation: (for beginners)

Stretch both legs straight in front of the body.
Lean backward, using the arms for support, and rest the top of the head on the floor. Arch the back and place both palms on the thighs or let them rest on the floor.

FORWARD BENDING ASANAS

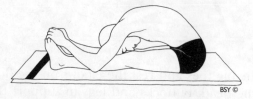

Paschimottanasana (back stretching pose)

Sit on the floor with the legs outstretched, feet together and hands on the knees.

This is the starting position.

Slowly bend forward from the hips, sliding the hands down the legs.

Try to grasp the big toes with the fingers and thumbs; or hold the heels, ankles or any part of the legs that can be reached comfortably.

Hold the position for a few seconds. Relax the back and leg muscles allowing them to gently stretch.

Keeping the legs straight and utilising the arm muscles, not the back muscles, begin to bend the elbows and gently bring the trunk down towards the legs, maintaining a firm grip on the toes, feet or legs.

Try to touch the knees with the forehead.

Do not strain.

This is the final position.

Hold the position for as long as is comfortable and relax.

Slowly return to the starting position.

This is one round.

Breathing: Inhale in the starting position.

Exhale slowly while bending forward.

Inhale in the static position.

Exhale while bringing the trunk further towards the legs with the arms.

Breathe slowly and deeply in the final position or retain the breath out if holding for a short duration.

Inhale while returning to the starting position.

Duration: Beginners should perform up to 5 rounds, remaining in the final position for only a short length of time. Adepts may maintain the final position for up to 5 minutes.

Contra-indications: People who suffer from slipped disc or sciatica should not practise paschimottanasana.

Pada Hastasana (forward bending pose)

Stand with the spine erect, feet together and hands beside the body. Distribute the weight of the body evenly on both feet. This is the starting position. Keep both the legs straight throughout the practice. Slowly bend forward, first bending the head, taking the chin towards the chest, then bending the upper trunk, relaxing the shoulders for- 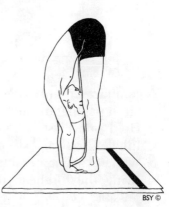 ward and letting the arms go limp. Bend the mid-trunk and finally the lower trunk.

While bending forward, imagine that the body has no bones or muscles. Bring the palms to the floor beside the feet. If this is not possible, bring the fingertips as near to the floor as possible. Bring the forehead towards the knees.

Hold the position, relaxing the whole back.

Slowly return to the starting position in the reverse order. This completes one round. Relax in the upright position before continuing the next round.

Breathing: Inhale in the starting position.
Exhale while bending forward.
Breathe slowly and deeply in the final position.
Inhale while returning to the starting position.

Duration: Practise up to 5 rounds, gradually increasing the time for which the posture is held and decreasing the

155

number of rounds, or practise one round for 3 to 5 minutes.

Contra-indications: This asana should not be practised by those people suffering from serious back complaints, sciatica, heart disease, high blood pressure or abdominal hernia.

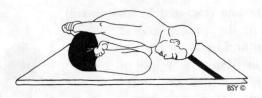

Yogamudrasana (psychic union pose)

Sit in padmasana and close the eyes.

Hold one wrist behind the back with the other hand.
Inhale slowly and deeply.

While exhaling bend forward keeping the spine straight.
Bring the forehead down to the floor or as close as possible.

Relax the whole body in the final position, breathing slowly and deeply.

Stay in the final position for as long as is comfortable without straining.

While inhaling slowly return to the starting position.

Repeat the pose with the legs crossed the other way around.

Duration: Try to remain in the final position for one or two minutes.

Contra-indications: People with serious eye, heart or back conditions should not attempt this asana.

Variation: for beginners

For those who are stiff and cannot touch the floor with their foreheads, instead of remaining in the final position, the body is raised and lowered a number of times.

156

SPINAL TWISTING ASANAS

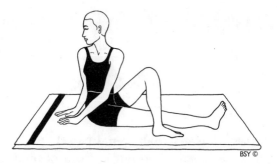

Meru Wakrasana (spinal twist)

Sit with the legs outstretched.

Turn the trunk slightly to the right and place the right hand behind the body, close to the left buttock, with the fingers pointing backward.

Place the left hand behind and slightly to the side of the right buttock.

Bend the left knee and place the foot outside the right knee.

Keeping the spine upright and straight, twist the head and trunk as far to the right as is comfortable, using the arms as levers. Look over the right shoulder as far as possible.

The buttocks should remain on the floor. The right elbow may bend a little.

Hold the final position.

Re-centre the trunk, relax for a few seconds and then twist again.

Practise up to 5 times and then repeat on the other side.

Breathing: Inhale before twisting.

Retain the breath inside while twisting.

Exhale while re-centring.

Contra-indications: People with severe back conditions, ulcers, hernias or other complaints of this nature, should not perform this asana.

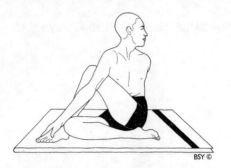

Ardha Matsyendrasana (half spinal twist)

Sit with the legs stretched out in front of the body.

Bend the right leg and place the right foot flat on the floor on the outside of the left knee.

Bend the left leg and bring the foot around to the right buttock.

Pass the left arm through the space between the chest and the right knee, and place it against the outside of the right leg.

Hold the right foot or ankle with the left hand, so that the right knee is close to the left armpit.

Sit up as straight as possible.

Slowly twist to the right Use the left arm as a lever against the right leg to twist the trunk as far as possible without using the back muscles.

Look over the right shoulder keeping the head level.

Bend the right elbow and place the arm around the back of the left side of the waist.

Breathing: Inhale in the forward position.

Exhale while twisting the trunk.

Breathe deeply and slowly without strain in the final position. Inhale while returning to the starting position.

Duration: Practise once on each side, gradually increasing the holding time to 1 or 2 minutes on each side of the body or up to 30 breaths.

Contra-indications: People suffering from peptic ulcer, hernia or hyperthyroidism should only practise this pose under expert guidance.

People with sciatica or slipped disc may benefit from the variation of this asana, but great care should be taken.

Variation: For beginners and those with stiff bodies, the leg that is placed by the side of the buttock should remain straight and the hand holding the ankle may be wrapped around the opposite thigh, hugging the knee to the chest.

INVERTED ASANAS

Always practise these asanas on a folded blanket thick enough to protect the vertebrae of the neck and back of the head. Never practise on a soft mattress, spring bed or air cushion. Shavasana should always follow an inverted asana.

Vipareeta Karani Asana (inverted pose)

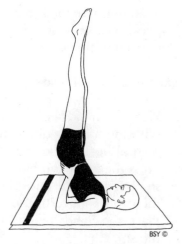

Lie flat on the back with the legs and feet together, arms by the side palms down.

Raise both legs, keeping them straight and together. Move the legs over the body towards the head.

Push down on the arms and hands, raising the buttocks. Roll the spine from the floor, taking the legs further over the head.

Turn the palms up, bend the elbows and let the top of the hips rest on the base of the palms near the wrist. Keep the elbows close together.

Raise both the legs to the vertical position and relax the feet.

In the final position, the trunk is at a 45 degree angle to the floor.

159

Close the eyes and relax in the final pose for as long as is comfortable.

To return to the starting position, lower the legs over the head, then place the hands on the floor, palms down.

Slowly lower the spine, vertebra by vertebra, along the floor.

When the buttocks reach the floor, lower the legs, keeping them straight.

Relax the body in shavasana.

Breathing: Inhale while in the lying position.

Retain the breath inside while assuming the final pose.

Once the body is steady in the final pose, practise normal or ujjayi breathing.

Retain the breath inside while lowering the body to the floor.

Duration: Beginners should practise for a few seconds only, gradually increasing the time over a period of weeks to an optimum of 3 to 5 minutes. This practice should be performed only once during the asana programme.

Contra-indications: As for sarvangasana.

Sarvangasana (shoulder stand pose)

Lie on the back on a folded blanket.

Place the hands beside the body palms down.

With the support of the arms, slowly raise the legs to the vertical position, keeping them straight.

Press the arms and hands down on the floor. Slowly and smoothly roll the buttocks and spine off the floor, raising the trunk to a vertical position.

Place the hands behind the ribcage, slightly away from the spine.

Gently push the chest forward so that it presses firmly against the chin.

In the final position, the legs are vertical, together and in a straight line with the trunk. The feet are relaxed.

Close the eyes. Relax the whole body in the final pose for as long as is comfortable.

To return to the starting position, bring the legs forward until the feet are above and behind the back of the head.

Keep the legs straight.

Release the position of the hands and place the arms on the floor, palms down.

Gradually lower the spine to the floor, followed by the buttocks, until the legs resume their initial vertical position.

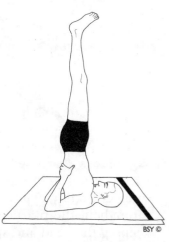

Slowly lower the legs to the floor.

Relax in shavasana until the respiration and heartbeat return to normal.

Breathing: Inhale in the starting position.

Retain the breath inside while assuming the final pose.

Practise slow, deep abdominal breathing in the final pose when the body is steady.

Retain the breath inside while lowering the body to the floor.

Duration: Beginners should hold the final position for a few seconds only, gradually increasing the time over a period of weeks to an optimum of 3 to 5 minutes. This practice should be performed only once during the asana programme.

Contra-indications: This asana should not be practised by people suffering from enlarged thyroid, liver or spleen, cervical spondylitis, slipped disc, high blood pressure or other heart ailments, weak blood vessels in the eyes, thrombosis or impure blood. It should be avoided during menstruation and advanced stages of pregnancy.

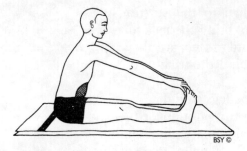

Tadagi Mudra (barrelled abdomen technique)

Sit with the legs stretched out in front of the body and the feet slightly apart. The legs should remain straight throughout the practice. Place the hands on the knees, keeping the head and spine straight.

Lean forward and grasp the big toes with the thumbs, index and second fingers, keeping the head facing forward.

Inhale slowly and deeply, expanding the abdominal muscles to their fullest extent.

Retain the breath inside for a comfortable length of time without straining.

Exhale slowly and deeply while relaxing the abdomen.

Maintain the hold on the toes.

Repeat the breathing up to 10 times.

Then release the toes and return to the starting position. This is 1 round.

Duration: Practise 3 to 5 rounds.

Contra-indications: Pregnant women and those suffering from hernia or prolapse should avoid this practice.

Practice note: Release the hold on the toes between breaths if the position becomes uncomfortable.

23

Pranayama

Prana is the vital force that pervades the whole cosmos. It is in all things and it is the bioenergy that activates the human organism. It is closely related to the air that we breathe, which is our main source of prana. However, the air is only the vehicle, it is not prana itself. Prana is the medium that links body and soul. It is the connecting force between consciousness and matter and can be regarded as a very subtle aspect of both matter and physical energy.

Yama means control. Thus pranayama is a series of techniques that aim at stimulating and increasing the vital energy in the body by directing it to particular areas for special purposes, including healing. Pranayama ensures that the flow of vital energy in the body is free and unimpeded, helping to maintain good health.

Pranayama, correctly used, is the bridge between body and mind. It should be performed gently and with awareness. It should never be forced in the expectation of better results, as this is a block to success. It is better to practise below your maximum capacity at first so that you do not suffer strain.

Pranayama also brings tranquillity and restricts interference from the thought process. It stills the disturbances of the mind, freeing us to tune into the subtle aspect of our being. Pranayama is therefore a vital technique for all those who follow the spiritual path.

The following points should be carefully read and carried out before starting to do pranayama:

- The bladder, stomach and intestines should be empty before doing pranayama. Wait for at least four hours after meals.
- Do pranayama after asana but before meditation practices.
- While doing pranayama, the body should be relaxed as much as possible. The spine, neck and head should be erect and centred.
- During pranayama there should be no strain. Breath retention must not be done for longer than is comfortable. This is most important as the lungs are very delicate organs and any misuse can lead to injury.
- Practise in a well ventilated (not windy), clean and pleasant environment.
- When beginning pranayama, some constipation and a reduction in the quantity of urine expelled may be experienced. In the case of dry motions stop taking salt or spices. If you have loose motions stop pranayama for a few days and take to a diet of rice and curd (yoghurt).
- Cover the body with a comfortable garment, sheet or blanket so that there are no external disturbances, such as insects, during the practices.
- Pranayama should not be practised during illness, although simple techniques such as breath awareness and abdominal breathing in shavasana may be performed. Always consult a yoga therapist or teacher before using any pranayama for therapeutic purposes.

Abdominal (or diaphragmatic) breathing

Lie in shavasana and relax the whole body. Observe the spontaneous breath without controlling it in any way. Continue observing the natural breath for some time.

Place the right hand on the abdomen just above the navel and the left hand on the centre of the chest.

Slowly inhale and expand the abdomen as much as possible.

164

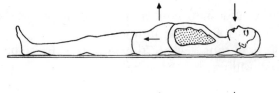

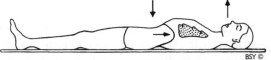

BSY ©

Slowly exhale while contracting the abdomen.
Try not to move the chest or shoulders.
The right hand moves up with inhalation and down with exhalation.
The left hand should not move with the breath.
Continue breathing slowly and deeply.
At the end of the inhalation the navel will be at its highest point.
On exhalation the navel moves downward towards the spine.
Continue for a few minutes.

Yogic breathing

Sit in a meditation posture or lie in shavasana and relax the whole body.
Inhale slowly and deeply, allowing the abdomen to expand fully.
At the end of abdominal expansion, as the inhalation continues start to expand the chest outward and upward. When the ribs are fully expanded, inhale a little more until expansion is felt in the clavicular area, the upper portion of the lungs around the base of the neck.
This completes one inhalation. The whole process should be one continuous movement.
Now start to exhale.
First, relax the clavicular area in the upper part of the chest; then allow the chest to contract downward and then inward.

Next, the abdomen contracts as the diaphragm pushes upward and toward the lungs.

Without straining, empty the lungs by drawing the abdominal wall toward the spine.

The entire breath movement should be harmonious and flowing.

Hold the breath for a few seconds at the end of exhalation. This completes one round of yogic breathing.

At first perform 5 to 10 rounds and slowly increase to 10 minutes daily.

Practice note: Once control of the breathing process has been established, the clavicular technique is dropped and yogic breathing is modified to become a combination of abdominal and thoracic breathing.

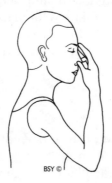

Hand position: Nasagra Mudra (nosetip position)

Hold the fingers of the right hand in front of the face.

Rest the index and middle fingers gently on the eyebrow centre.

The thumb is above the right nostril and the ring finger above the left.

These two digits control the flow of breath in the nostrils by alternately pressing on one nostril, blocking the flow of breath, and then the other.

When practising for long periods, the left hand may support the right elbow.

Nadi Shodhana Pranayama (psychic network purification)
Technique 1: Preparatory practice

Sit in any comfortable meditation posture. Keep the head and spine upright.

Relax the whole body and close the eyes.

Practise yogic breathing for some time.

Adopt nasagra mudra with the right hand and place the left hand on the knee.

Close the right nostril with the thumb.

Inhale and exhale through the left nostril 5 times.

The rate of inhalation/exhalation should be normal.

After 5 breaths release the pressure of the thumb on the right nostril and close the left nostril with the ring finger.

Inhale and exhale through the right nostril 5 times, keeping the respiration rate normal.

Lower the hand and breathe 5 times through both nostrils together.

This is one round.

Practise 5 rounds or for 3 to 5 minutes, making sure that there is no sound as the air passes through the nostrils.

After practising for 15 days go on to technique 2.

Technique 2: Alternate nostril breathing

In this technique the duration of inhalation/exhalation is controlled.

Close the right nostril with the thumb and breathe in using yogic breathing through the left nostril.

At the same time count mentally, "1, Om; 2, Om; 3, Om", until the inhalation ends comfortably. This is the basic count.

Close the left nostril with the ring finger, release the pressure of the thumb on the right nostril and breathe out through the right nostril, making the same count.

The time for inhalation and exhalation should be equal, a ratio of 1:1.

Next, inhale through the right nostril, keeping the same count.

167

At the end of inhalation close the right nostril, open the left nostril and exhale through the left nostril, counting as before.

This is one round.

Practise 5 rounds.

Ratio and timing: After a few days, if there is no difficulty, increase the length of inhalation/exhalation by one count keeping the same ratio. Continue in this way, increasing the inhalation/exhalation by one count as it becomes easy.

After perfecting the above ratio, it may be changed to 1:2. For example, breathe in for a count of 5 and breathe out for a count of 10. Continue extending the breath by adding one count to the inhalation and two to the exhalation. When this technique can be performed with complete ease move on to technique 3.

Technique 3: with Antar Kumbhaka (inner retention)

In this technique antar kumbhaka or internal breath retention is introduced.

Close the right nostril and breathe in slowly through the left nostril for a count of 5.

At the end of inhalation, close both nostrils and retain the breath for a count of 5.

Open the right nostril, breathe in slightly through the right nostril and then slowly breathe out through the same nostril for a count of 5.

At the end of exhalation, immediately inhale through the right nostril for a count of 5, keeping the left nostril closed.

Again, retain the breath for a count of 5 with both nostrils closed.

Open the left nostril, breathe in slightly through the left nostril and then breathe out through the same nostril for a count of 5.

This is one round using a ratio of 1:1:1.

Practise 5 rounds.

Ratio and timing: The maintenance of a strict ratio during inhalation, kumbhaka and exhalation is important. After mastering the ratio of 1:1:1, increase the ratio to 1:1:2. For example, inhale for a count of 5, perform internal kumbhaka for a count of 5 and exhale for a count of 10. After some weeks of practice, when this ratio has been mastered, increase the ratio to 1:2:2. Inhale for a count of 5, do internal kumbhaka for a count of 10 and exhale for a count of 10.

After mastering the ratio of 1:2:2, gradually increase the count by adding one unit to the inhalation, 2 units to the retention and 2 units to the exhalation. The count of one round will then be 6:12:12.

Advanced practice: Nadi shodhana pranayama may be practised in conjunction with jalandhara and moola bandhas. First practise only jalandhara bandha during internal breath retention. Once this practice has been perfected then introduce moola bandha with jalandhara during internal retention

Duration: 5 rounds daily.

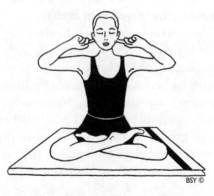

Bhramari Pranayama (humming bee breath)
Sit in a comfortable meditation asana with the hands resting on the knees.
Close the eyes and feel the whole body becoming quiet and steady.

169

The lips should remain gently closed with the jaw relaxed and the teeth slightly separated throughout the practice.

Raise the arms sideways, bringing the hands to the ears.

Use the index or middle finger to plug the ears.

Breathe in through the nose.

Exhale slowly and in a controlled manner while making a deep, steady humming sound like that of the black bee.

The humming sound should be smooth, even and continuous for the duration of the exhalation.

The sound should be soft and mellow.

Become aware of the vibration created by the sound inside the head.

This is one round. At the end of exhalation, breathe in deeply and repeat the process.

Perform 5 rounds.

Duration: Practise 5 to 10 rounds in the beginning, then slowly increase to 10 to 15 minutes.

Time of practice: The best time to practise is late at night or in the early morning. However, bhramari may be practised at any time to relieve mental tension.

Ujjayi Pranayama (the psychic breath)

Sit in any comfortable position, preferably a meditation asana. Close the eyes and relax the whole body.

Take the awareness to the breath in the nostrils and allow the breathing to become calm and rhythmic.

After some time, transfer the awareness to the throat.

Try to feel or imagine that the breath is being drawn in and out through the throat and not through the nostrils.

Gently contract the glottis so that a soft snoring sound like the breathing of a sleeping baby is produced in the throat.

Practise abdominal breathing. Both inhalation and exhalation should be long and even and at the same time relaxed.

Concentrate on the sound produced by the breath in the throat. The sound of the breath should not be very loud.

It should just be audible to the practitioner.

When this has been mastered, the tongue can be folded back into khechari mudra, so that the lower surface lies in contact with the upper palate. Stretch the tip of the tongue as far back as is comfortable.

Duration: Practise for 10 to 20 minutes.

Contra-indications: People who are too introverted by nature should not perform this practice.

Practice note: Ujjayi may be performed in any position, standing, sitting or lying, except when practised with khechari mudra, which should be done in a sitting position.

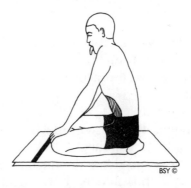

Preparatory practice: Swana Pranayama (panting breath)

Sit in vajrasana and separate the knees as far as is possible, keeping the big toes in contact. Place the hands on the knees and close the eyes.

Straighten the arms and lean forward slightly. Keep the head erect.

Open the mouth wide and extend the tongue outside.

Breathe through the mouth in a manner that resembles the panting of a dog.

While breathing out the abdomen should contract and while breathing in the abdomen should expand. Keep the chest as still as possible.

The breathing should be passive, only occurring because of the movement of the abdomen.

171

Breathe in and out 10 to 20 times.
This is one round. Relax and breathe normally before starting the next round.

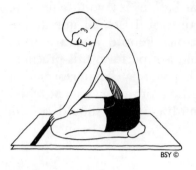

Agnisar Kriya (activating the digestive fire or cleansing with the essence of fire)
This technique may be practised in the same position or in padmasana.
Breathe in deeply.
Exhale, emptying the lungs as much as possible.
Perform jalandhara bandha.
Contract and expand the abdominal muscles rapidly for as long as it is possible to hold the breath outside comfortably.
Release jalandhara bandha.
When the head is upright take a slow, deep breath in.
This is one round. Relax until the breathing normalises before commencing the next round.

Duration: Three rounds of 10 abdominal contractions and expansions is sufficient at first. With regular practice, the number of abdominal movements may be increased over a period of time.

Contra-indications: People suffering from high blood pressure, heart disease, acute duodenal or peptic ulcers, overactive thyroid gland or chronic diarrhoea should not perform this kriya. Women who are pregnant should not practise.

Bhastrika Pranayama (bellows breath)

Sit in any comfortable meditation posture with the hands on the knees.

Raise the right hand and perform nasagra mudra.

Left nostril: Close the right nostril with the thumb.

Breathe in and out forcefully, without straining, through the left nostril 10 times. Count each breath mentally. The abdomen should expand and contract rhythmically with the breath in a pumping action.

Do not expand the chest or raise the shoulders. The body should not jerk.

After 10 respirations, breathe in deeply through the left nostril keeping the right nostril closed.

Close both nostrils and hold the breath inside for a few seconds.

Exhale through the left nostril.

Right nostril: Close the left nostril and perform the same practice in the same way in the right nostril.

After 10 respirations, breathe in deeply through the right nostril keeping the left nostril closed.

Close both nostrils and hold the breath inside for a few seconds.

Exhale through the right nostril.

Both nostrils: Open both nostrils bringing the right hand to the knee and perform the same practice in the same way through both nostrils.

After 10 respirations, breathe in deeply through both nostrils.

Close both nostrils and hold the breath inside for a few seconds.

Exhale through both nostrils.

Breathing through the left, the right and both nostrils, as above, forms one complete round.

Breathing: Bhastrika may be practised at three different breath rates: slow (one breath every two seconds), medium (one breath every second) and fast (two breaths per second), depending on the capacity of the practitioner.

Beginners are advised to start with the slow rate until proficient, then increase the rate.

The number of breaths may be increased by 5 per month to a maximum of 40 to 50 through the left, right and both nostrils.

Duration: Up to 5 rounds. Slowly increase the duration of retention up to 30 seconds after breathing through the left, the right and both nostrils. Do not strain.

Precautions: A feeling of faintness, excessive perspiration or a vomiting sensation indicates that the practice is being performed incorrectly. Stop the practice and seek the advice of a yoga teacher. Beginners are advised to take a short rest after each round.

Contra-indications: Bhastrika should not be practised by people who suffer from high blood pressure, heart disease, hernia, gastric ulcer, stroke, epilepsy or vertigo. Those suffering from lung diseases such as asthma and chronic bronchitis, or who are recovering from tuberculosis, are recommended to practise only under expert guidance.

Kapalbhati Pranayama (frontal brain cleansing breath)

Sit in any comfortable meditation asana with the hands resting on the knees.

Close the eyes and relax the whole body.

Inhale through both nostrils, expanding the abdomen, and exhale with a forceful contraction of the abdominal muscles. Do not strain.

The next inhalation takes place by passively allowing the abdominal muscles to expand. Inhalation should be a spontaneous or passive recoil, involving no effort.

Perform 10 respirations to begin with. Count each respiration mentally.

After completing 10 rapid breaths in succession, inhale and exhale deeply.

This is one round. Practise 3 to 5 rounds.

After completing the practice, maintain awareness of the region of the eyebrow centre.

174

Breathing: It is important that the rapid breathing used in these techniques be from the abdomen and not from the chest.

The number of respirations may be increased from the initial count of 10 up to 20, as the abdominal muscles become stronger.

Duration: Up to 5 rounds of 10 to 20 breaths.

Precautions: If pain or dizziness is experienced, stop the practice. If the problem continues, consult a yoga teacher.

Contra-indications: Kapalbhati should not be practised by those suffering from heart disease, high blood pressure, vertigo, epilepsy, stroke, hernia or gastric ulcer.

24

Bandhas

Bandhas are the physical techniques that allow the practitioner to control the different organs and nerves of the body, and they constitute a very important group of practices. During the performance of bandhas various parts of the body are contracted or tightened, massaging the internal organs and their nerves and blood vessels.

It has been scientifically demonstrated that in normal people bandhas help to maintain equilibrium in the blood pressure. They do this by increasing the flow of blood in the peripheral blood vessels, and thereby they decrease sympathetic nervous stimulation and increase para-sympathetic stimulation at the central nervous system level. They also increase the size of the entrance to the chest and chest cavity, facilitating healthy breathing. However, this does not apply to people who have high blood pressure; they should seek advice from their yoga teacher before practising bandhas.

In terms of asthma and diabetes the relevance of these findings is obvious. The decrease in sympathetic nervous system stimulation is beneficial to all the illnesses discussed in this book, as it brings about a rebalancing of the autonomic nervous system and a reduction of the effects of stress on the body.

Bandhas also have a certain psychic effect through their influence on the chakras. They help to redirect prana and

176

thereby ensure the free flow of healing energies in the body. When combined with pranayama, bandhas are extremely powerful techniques, which promote good health through the change in the subtle qualities within.

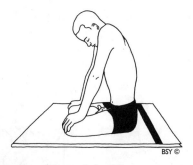

Jalandhara Bandha (throat lock)

Sit in padmasana or siddha/siddha yoni asana with the head and spine straight. The knees should be in firm contact with the floor.

Those who cannot manage this may perform jalandhara bandha in a standing position.

Place the palms of the hands on the knees. Close the eyes and relax.

Inhale slowly and deeply, and retain the breath inside.

While retaining the breath, bend the head forward and press the chin tightly against the chest.

Straighten and lock the arms, pressing the knees down with the hands.

Simultaneously, hunch the shoulders upward and forward.

Stay in the final position for as long as the breath can be held comfortably.

Relax the shoulders, bend the arms, slowly release the lock, raise the head and then exhale.

Repeat when the respiration has returned to normal.

Breathing: The practice may also be performed with external breath retention.

Duration: This practice may be repeated up to 5 times.

177

Contra-indications: People suffering from cervical spondy-losis, high intracranial pressure, vertigo, high blood pressure or heart disease should not practise jalandhara bandha.

Practice note: Do not inhale or exhale until the chin lock and arm lock have been released and the head is fully upright.

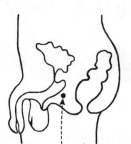 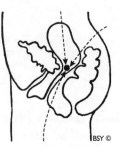

Fig. 1: For the male   Fig. 2: For the female

Technique 1: Moola Bandha (perineum contraction)

Sit in siddha/siddha yoni asana so that pressure is applied to the perineal/vaginal region.

Close the eyes and relax.

Be aware of the natural breath for a short while.

Then focus the awareness on the perineal/vaginal region. Contract this region by pulling up on the muscles of the pelvic floor and then relaxing them.

Continue to briefly contract and relax the perineal/vaginal region as rhythmically and evenly as possible.

Technique 2: Moola Bandha with internal breath retention

Sit in siddha/siddha yoni asana. Place the palms on the knees. Close the eyes and relax.

Inhale deeply, retain the breath inside and perform jalandhara bandha.

Maintaining jalandhara, perform moola bandha by slowly contracting the perineal/vaginal region and holding the contraction. Do not strain. This is the final lock.

178

Hold it for as long as the breath can comfortably be retained.

Slowly release moola bandha, release jalandhara bandha, raise the head to the upright position, and exhale.

Practise up to 10 times.

Contra-indications: This practice should only be performed under the guidance of an experienced yoga teacher.

Practice note: Moola bandha is the contraction of certain muscles in the pelvic floor. In the male body the area of contraction lies between the anus and the testes. In the female body, the point of contraction is behind the cervix.

25

Meditation

Yogic experience over the centuries has established that meditation is a powerful force in removing disease, and today scientific research is detailing the profound and wide ranging contribution of meditation towards optimum good health. Laboratory tests have shown that meditation has the following effects on the body:

- Decreases oxygen consumption (indicating relaxation and more efficient respiration).
- Lowers blood pressure.
- Relaxes the sympathetic nervous system, resulting in lower levels of the 'stress hormones' adrenaline and noradrenaline.
- Increases electrical skin resistance (an index of relaxation).
- Cuts production and build-up of lactic acid.
- Slows brain rhythms to the alpha level, indicating relaxed awareness and the absence of stress.
- Slows the heart rate.
- Decreases carbon dioxide production.

Effects that can be monitored by scientific instruments are just a few of those that occur during meditation, yet each of these physiological changes has a positive influence on health.

The effects of meditation on the mind and states of consciousness are measured on alpha wave monitors, which have been used in many tests including those where patients made use of mantras to lower their blood pressure. Such tests show that meditation leads to the predominance of alpha waves in the brain, especially the frontal and central areas. Alpha waves range from eight to thirteen cycles per second, but in meditation only the slower waves of eight to nine cycles per second are usually recorded, indicating very deep states of relaxation. There is also an increase in theta wave activity, which is associated in sleep with dreaming, and at other times with the experience of creative inspiration, a joyful state that invigorates the body and spirit alike.

Documentation of effects such as these have led to meditation becoming increasingly accepted by the international medical fraternity as a valuable aid in overcoming disease, to the extent that researchers in the United States have even incorporated meditation in the treatment of cancer.

Through meditation, many of the unconscious nervous functions of the human organism can be brought under conscious control, and managed so as to balance the mental and physical energies. By learning to balance the involuntary nervous system we are no longer dominated by the stress and strain of modern living, and the mind/body complex is thus less susceptible to illness.

There are hundreds of yogic practices for turning from the distractions of the external world and 'going in' to experience the healing relaxation that so profoundly affects the body, mind and soul. However, included in this section are only those techniques that are most relevant to people suffering from asthma and diabetes. In the process of eliminating their illness, they will also find that, at the same time, these techniques are most valuable in expanding awareness and approaching the higher self.

RELAXATION

Relaxation is not just sinking into an armchair, not being able to move. It is a dynamic vitality which pervades every moment and aspect of living and it makes us more capable of acting efficiently and joyfully. We may be more relaxed working hard than just sitting exhausted, taking it easy.

The relaxation exercise here removes all three kinds of tension – muscular, emotional, and psychic – thus removing the pranic blocks that manifest ultimately as asthma or diabetes. It may be practised any time you feel tired, tense or sick and it will refresh both body and mind. It is also ideally practised before bed in order to cut the repetitive chatter of the day's thoughts and worries and ensures a restful, healing sleep. This practice is also an ideal preparation for meditation.

Stage 1: Preparation

Lie down in shavasana. Adjust your position so that you feel the least possible discomfort.

Close your eyes and relax yourself completely.

Become aware of the whole body.

Feel that the body is part of the ground.

Feel all the sensations of the body and, if possible, try to create a mental image of the body.

Be aware of any aches or pains.

Direct your awareness to the source of this discomfort and try to be aware of nothing else.

Let this pain be a focus for your awareness; this will not be difficult.

If your mind starts to wander, let it.

But simultaneously try to maintain your awareness of the pain in the body.

Continue for a few minutes.

Stage 2: Body awareness

Then direct your awareness to the right foot.

Be aware of nothing else but the right foot.

After a short time, transfer your awareness to the left foot. You can create a mental picture of the left foot or feel the sensations connected with it. Whatever, continue to be aware.

Transfer your awareness to the right leg and repeat the process.

Repeat the same thing in turn with the left leg, the abdomen, chest, right arm, left arm, neck, head and finally, the whole body.

This is one round.

Intensify your awareness as much as possible.

Even though your awareness may stray onto other subjects, continue to be aware of the body.

Do another round, beginning with the right foot again. Remain aware.

Move your awareness through the different parts of the body. Try to feel the different parts of the body as you have never felt them before.

Continue your practice in this way.

Stage 3: Breath awareness

This can be practised as a continuation of stages 1 and 2 or as a separate practice. Close your eyes, or keep the eyes closed. Become aware of your breathing.

Imagine that you are breathing in and out from the abdomen. Breathe directly from the abdomen.

You must count each breath from fifteen back to zero.

As you inhale, count fifteen. As you exhale count fifteen. As you inhale again, count fourteen. As you exhale count fourteen and so on.

Continue in this way to zero, maintaining awareness of the breathing process and mental counting.

Your breath should be natural.

If you lose count, start again, each time you lose count.

Then, move the awareness to the chest and imagine that each inhalation and exhalation moves in and out at the heart.

Count each inhalation and exhalation from fifteen back to zero as before (at the abdomen).

Now, move the awareness to the throat and imagine that each inhalation and exhalation move in and out at the throat.

Count each inhalation and exhalation from fifteen back to zero as before.

Now, be aware of the flow of breath through the nostrils, carefully noting all sensations. Count the breaths in the same way as before. Maintain awareness of the flow of breath through nostrils and mental counting.

End the practice when you are ready by letting go of breath awareness, becoming aware of the body, then externalizing the awareness and slowly coming out of shavasana.

AJAPA JAPA

Japa is the constant repetition of mantra. Japa becomes ajapa (spontaneous) when the mantra repeats itself automatically, without conscious effort. This technique uses the spontaneous mantra of the breath, *soham*, to calm the mind and to transfer this mental tranquillity to the body, effecting healing at the deepest level of being.

Awakening prana in the frontal psychic passage and in the spinal cord rebalances the body, increases energy and purifies the mind so that the whole organism functions at a healthier, more efficient level.

Practice note

During the preliminary practice of ajapa japa, the practitioner should try to feel the prana (healing bioenergy) flowing in the frontal psychic passage that runs between the navel and the throat. Your teacher will help you locate this passage. In the beginning you will need to use your imagination, but later this pranic passage will become a definite reality.

Technique 2 follows exactly the same stages and manner of practice as technique 1, but instead of moving between the navel and throat, the awareness moves in the spinal column. The awareness ascends in the spinal column with inhalation and descends with exhalation, between mooladhara chakra (a point at the perineum in the male body, or the cervix in the female body) and ajna chakra (a point inside the head behind the eyebrow centre).

184

Technique 1: Frontal passage rotation
Stage 1: Soham

Sit in a comfortable position. Close your eyes and relax the whole body. Hold the spine upright, without strain.

Tell yourself that for the duration of the practice all problems and worries will be discarded, all attention will only be on the practice of ajapa japa.

Become aware of your breathing process.

As you breathe in, know that you are breathing in.

When breathing out, know you are breathing out.

Be totally attentive to every incoming and outgoing breath; feel the rhythm of the flow.

Carry on in this manner for a few minutes.

Then imagine that the breath is flowing between the navel and the front of the throat.

On inhalation, the breath rises from the navel to the throat.

On exhalation, the breath descends from the throat to navel.

At first you may find this process a little difficult to imagine, but be patient. The important thing is to be completely aware of the breath.

Let the breathing become rhythmical, deep and long, but without force. The more you relax, the more the breath will automatically become slow and deep.

Continue in this manner for five minutes. Maintain awareness. If the mind wanders, which it probably will, don't fight it, but try to maintain breath awareness.

Then you must merge and synchronize the mantra *soham* with the breath. You must be simultaneously aware of both the ascending and descending breath and the sound *soham* made at the throat.

Mantra and breath must be synchronized so that the *so* sounds with the upward moving inhalation and the *ham* sounds with the downward moving exhalation.

There should be unceasing awareness of *soham* as you breathe in and out between the navel and the throat.

If your mind wanders, let it, but be aware that it is wandering. Maintain mantra and breath awareness.

Continue in this manner for the length of the time that you have assigned for the practice.

Stage 2: Hamso

This is exactly the same practice as in stage 1 but now with an emphasis on *hamso*.

Ham is still the downward moving exhalation and *so* is still the upward moving inhalation, but the emphasis is reversed.

Start with exhalation – *ham*. Finish with inhalation – *so*.

There should be no pause between *ham* and *so*, but a slight pause after one round of *hamso*. That is, there should be no pause between exhalation and inhalation but a slight pause at the end of inhalation just before exhaling.

Stage 3: Frontal passage rotation with ujjayi and khechari

This is exactly the same practice as in stage 1, but now done in conjunction with ujjayi pranayama and khechari mudra. (Roll the tongue backwards so that the normally lower surface touches the upper palate. Try to bring the tongue back on the roof of the mouth as far as possible without strain.)

After some time, practise *hamso* as in stage 2

Technique 2: Spinal passage rotation

Stage 1: Soham

Practise *soham* (as in technique 1, stage 1) but with the awareness in the spinal column – *So* ascending with inhalation and *ham* descending with exhalation

Stage 2: Hamso

Then, practise *hamso* (as in technique 1, stage 2), still with the awareness in the spinal column.

Stage 3: Spinal passage rotation with ujjayi and khechari

This is exactly the same as in stages 1 and 2, but now done in conjunction with ujjayi pranayama and khechari mudra.

YOGA NIDRA

Yoga nidra is a systematic method of inducing complete mental, physical and emotional relaxation. It is a state of relaxed awareness on the borderline between sleep and wakefulness, allowing contact with the subconscious and unconscious minds, while remaining awake and aware.

Yoga nidra is the yogic tranquillizer, the natural means to establish harmony and well-being through the entire system. It is a superbly effective system of meditation and, for people who are sick or weak, it rejuvenates the nervous system, awakening prana and great healing power. Yoga nidra is especially useful in overcoming psychosomatic diseases, and similar techniques are used in clinics and hospitals throughout the world.

This technique can be practised anywhere, at any time. However, the best place is a well-ventilated room with soft light and a comfortable temperature. Clothing should be minimal and very loose, and a light sheet might be necessary to protect the practitioner from the cold or insects. Privacy is essential and sudden interruptions should be avoided.

The best time to do yoga nidra is in the early evening, after bathing, before the evening meal. It can also be done in the early morning after some practice of asana and pranayama first, and during the day to help release accumulated tension. Practise yoga nidra just before sleeping if you have insomnia. Try to establish a regular time. Do not practise immediately after eating; allow at least two hours for digestion of a heavy meal and half an hour for the settling of light refreshments.

Yoga nidra is practised in the pose called shavasana, with head, trunk and limbs in one straight line. However, some people will prefer to use a thin pillow under the head and shoulders or under the small of the back.

During the practice you should aim to gain a grasp of the technique so that you can recall all the instructions without conscious efforts. It is recommended that you learn this technique from a yoga teacher, but if this is not possible,

187

you could put the instructions on tape or have someone read them to you.

Resolve

The resolve is a short, positive phrase repeated at the beginning and end of the practice of yoga nidra. It is a seed that is planted deep in the unconscious mind and can bring extraordinary results if used with sincerity and feeling. The resolve has great healing potential, planting a positive suggestion at a time when the unconscious mind is in the state of greatest receptivity. It should be short, to the point and deeply felt. Some people have found the following resolves very useful:
• I am attaining perfect health.
• I am becoming whole.
• I am unchanging consciousness, beyond disease.

You should continue to repeat your resolve, in exactly the same words, with a fervent and determined attitude, until it is a reality in your life.

Visualization

A most active area of the brain is the visual cortex, indicating that the brain is very receptive to visual imagery. This means that inner or mental visualization has powerful effects on the brain and thus the whole organism. In the following practice of yoga nidra we use this capacity for self-healing by giving specific visualizations for each of the illnesses discussed in this book. At first these visualizations will require the use of imagination, but with practice they will gain clarity and substance. As your awareness expands, you will not only move towards health but also start to take off into the realms of higher consciousness.

Alternative visualizations: The appropriate visualization may be inserted in the practice to replace the section 'healing symbols'. These visualizations are specifically directed at channelling the healing energies of the body.

188

Preparation: Get ready for yoga nidra. Lie in shavasana and make yourself as comfortable as possible. Keep your feet apart and left them flop a little sideways, arms close to the body, but not touching, with palms upwards. (*pause*) Adjust your blanket, clothes and position so that you can practise yoga nidra without moving and with no physical discomfort. Please close your eyes and keep them closed. (*long pause*)

The practice of yoga nidra is the act of hearing and act of feeling; these are the only important factors. (*pause*) In yoga nidra you function at the level of awareness...plus the level of listening. In dream you have no control, but in yoga nidra you are the creator of the dream. (*pause*) Say to yourself mentally "I will remain awake"...repeat to yourself "I will remain awake". (*pause*) Give yourself some time to become calm and steady...take a deep breath and as you breathe in feel calmness diffusing throughout the body. (*pause*) As you breathe out feel yourself letting go.

Become aware of sounds in the distance, be aware of the most distant sounds that you can hear. (*pause*) Let the sense of hearing operate like a radar beam...searching out distant sounds and following them for a few seconds. (*pause*) Move the awareness quickly from sound to sound...without attempting to identify the source. (*pause*) Gradually bring the awareness to closer sounds...to sounds outside this building...and then to sounds inside the building...(*pause*) Now develop your awareness of this room...without opening your eyes visualize the four walls, the ceiling, the floor, your body lying on the floor. (*pause*) Become aware of the existence of your physical body lying on the floor...total awareness of the body lying in perfect stillness. (*pause*) Your body lying on the floor... develop awareness of the meeting points between the body and the floor.

Now become aware of the natural breath...be aware of the natural, spontaneous breath. Do not try to concentrate, as this will interfere with the natural process. (*pause*) Just

189

be aware and know that you are breathing. (*pause*) The practice of yoga nidra begins now...repeat mentally to yourself: "I am going to practise yoga nidra. I will remain awake. I will remain aware. I am going to practise yoga nidra."

Resolve: This is the time to make your resolve. (*pause*) A simple resolve. Please state your resolve mentally with feeling and awareness three times. (*pause*) Let it be a positive goal for your whole being.

Rotation of consciousness: Rotation of consciousness through the different centres of the body...as quickly as possible your awareness is to move from point to point. Please repeat mentally the name of each part and simultaneously become aware of that part. The practice always begins with the right hand...

Right side: Right hand thumb, second finger, third finger, fourth finger, fifth finger, palm, wrist, elbow, shoulder, armpit, waist, hip, right thigh, knee, calf muscle, ankle, heel, sole, right big toe, second toe, third toe, fourth toe, fifth toe...

Left side: Left hand thumb, second finger, third finger, fourth finger, fifth finger, palm, wrist, elbow, shoulder, armpit, waist, hip, left thigh, knee, calf muscle, ankle, heel, sole, left big toe, second toe, third toe, fourth toe, fifth toe...

Back: Right shoulder, left shoulder, the right shoulder blade, the left shoulder blade...right buttock, left buttock, the spine...the whole of the back together...

Front: Top of the head, forehead, right eyebrow, left eyebrow, the space between the eyebrows, right eye, left eye, right ear, left ear, right cheek, left cheek, nose, tip of the nose, upper lip, lower lip, chin, throat, the right collarbone, left collarbone, right chest, left chest, middle of the chest, navel, abdomen, lower abdomen...

Major parts: Whole of the right leg, whole of the left leg, both legs together...whole of the right arm, whole of the left arm, both arms together...whole of the back, whole of the front, whole of the head...together...whole body...whole body...whole body. (*long pause*)

Breath awareness: Draw your attention to the ingoing and outgoing breath. (*pause*) Feel the breath move along the passage between the navel and the throat...on inhalation it rises from the navel to the throat, on exhalation it descends from the throat to the navel. (*pause*) Be completely aware of the respiration, navel to throat, throat to navel...do not try to force the breath...just awareness. (*pause*)

Now let go of the awareness between navel to throat. As you breathe in, feel the body expand, and as you breathe out feel the body relax...inhale and expand, filling the body with healing energy...exhale and relax, feeling the impurities flow out of your system on the breath. (*pause*) Inhale and expand as the prana flows to every cell and every fibre of the body...exhale and relax, washing away negativity and impurities. (*pause*) Remain awake and continue the practice. (*long pause*)

Visualization: Are you awake or sleeping? Check yourself and then say mentally "I am awake"...Become aware of manipura chakra, the psychic energy centre in the solar plexus region. Manipura chakra, in the spinal cord behind the navel...As you exhale, feel the vital energy in your body gathering in manipura chakra. (*pause*) Exhale and withdraw all your prana, all your healing life force, into manipura chakra. (*pause*) Then as you inhale, feel this healing energy streaming to all parts of your body. (*pause*) See prana as streaks of light converging on manipura as you exhale...then as you inhale, visualize this healing prana flaring out from manipura to all parts of your body, like golden, healing sunrays. See a brilliant, gold, fiery sun at your navel, pulsating with health giving energy. (*pause*) Just as from a charcoal fire you see sparks shooting out with a hissing noise, so you see the healing energies moving in your body...clearly see the luminous shafts of energy...like the iridescent light streaks streaming

191

forth from fireworks. (*pause*) Imagine manipura to be a storehouse of infinite light streaks... Like a volcano erupting light particles moving with white lightning speed...They permeate the whole body. (*pause*) Then the eruption stops and the lightning withdraws to the source, to reappear at the next explosion. (*long pause*)

Healing symbols: Take your awareness to chidakasha, the space you see in front of your closed eyes. (*pause*) In this space see a blue sky...a giant, golden sun...the warmth and golden energy of this sun...an explosion of light...a blue sky...a cross...a six-pointed star...a garden with a circular pool at the centre...in the pool a fountain...from the fountain a fine spray of golden, life giving liquid...blue lotus...white lotus...red lotus...shivalingam...candle flame...golden egg...stars at night...golden harvest moon...golden river...a sea of golden liquid...an endless golden ocean...See yourself at the edge of this ocean...you dive into the sea...feel it surround every part of your body...refreshing, tingling...soaking to the very depths of your being...recharging your body with vitality...smooth feeling. See yourself finding a shining, green jewel...Hold this sea emerald...gaze into the green jewel...It explodes in a blaze of light...and you find yourself on the shore. (*long pause*)

Inner space: Bring your awareness back to chidakasha, bring your awareness back to the dark space you see before your closed eyes. (*pause*) Watch the darkness that you see very carefully, with detachment; do not become involved. (*pause*) Rest your mind in this warm and friendly darkness...if any subtle phenomena manifest, for example, colours or patterns, simply take note of these and continue your awareness. (*pause*) If thoughts occur let them come and go, but continue to watch the dark space, continue this awareness. (*long pause*)

Resolve: Now the resolve, remember your resolve. Repeat the same resolve that you made at the beginning of the practice in the same words and with the same attitude.

Repeat your resolve with feeling and emphasis three times. (*pause*)

Finish: Become aware of the breathing, become aware of your natural breath. (*pause*) Awareness of breathing... and awareness of relaxation. (*pause*) Develop awareness of relaxation and awareness of your physical existence. (*pause*) Become aware of your arms and legs and of your whole physical body lying stretched out on the floor. (*pause*) Develop awareness of the room, walls, ceiling... noises in the room and noises outside. Bring your mind out...become completely external. (*pause*) Lie quietly for a few moments, keeping your eyes closed. Start moving your body, stretch yourself slowly...do not hurry. (*pause*) When you are sure that you are wide awake, sit up slowly and open your eyes. The practice of yoga nidra is now complete.

Hari Om Tat Sat

Alternative visualizations

For asthma: Now see the healing light extending into your nostrils, and your throat...As it travels you can feel its warmth and glowing quality...flowing smoothly down into the lungs...As you inhale see the breath carrying a stream of light sparks...on inhalation the stream of light sparks travel up into the nostril...down the throat...and into the lungs...On both sides of the lungs visualize the energy filling every inch of space...and pervading every cell...As it does so, see the mucus and stiffness of the lungs also being suffused with the golden sparks of light...Each particle of dried and hard mucus is now suffused with this life-giving force...Watch the energy dissolving mucus. (*pause*) As each piece of mucus in your lung dissolves, the energy moves deeper and deeper into the cell...The stiffness and rigidity of the tissues is broken down...the heat from this prana is dissolving the tissues...you can feel and see the gentle warmth of the light energy melting the lung tissue. (*pause*) The healing light is dissolving each and every part of your lungs right up through the bronchi and into the throat...slowly melting into a golden cast of your original lungs...you can see the impurities in the lungs being dissolved and melting into nothingness. (*pause*) Now the process reverses...the golden shape reforms into new tissue...help this process of rebuilding ...reform your lungs as you want them to be...strong lungs...elastic...whole...clean...healthy. (*pause*) Now see that your lungs have been reformed and are glowing with golden light. (*long pause*)

For diabetes: Now direct the golden light energy from manipura to the pancreas...be aware of your pancreas... against the back wall of your abdomen...just above the level of your navel...a long island of tissue. (*pause*) See the pancreas as an ocean of brilliant blue...dotted through this ocean are small green islands...you see them as if from a great height...each island produces insulin...but has not been functioning well until now. (*pause*) As you watch you see each island start to glow...a light deep within is illuminating the island. (*pause*) There are many green islands dotted through your blue ocean... each is now radiating prana...warmth and golden light. (*pause*) See the intensity of the light start to increase...the island start to pulsate with the intensity. (*pause*) Then each luminous island explodes...just like a volcano erupting ...throwing off impurities and blockages...and these impurities dissolve into nothingness...swallowed up by the blue ocean. (*pause*) Revealed to your vision is a molten inner core to each one of these islands...this golden core of warm and tingling energy has always been there but it was covered by impurities...now all the impurities are gone...all that remains is the pure essence of each island. (*pause*) Luminous golden islands in a deep blue ocean. (*pause*) Gradually the gold spreads into the sea as though from an infinite, radiant source...the whole ocean becomes golden...the whole pancreas becomes suffused with healing energy. (*pause*) As the intensity subsides, the pancreas and the islands are revealed, shining with golden light. (*long pause*)

Note: For full details of these practices consult the publications: *Asana Pranayama Mudra Bandha, Meditations from the Tantras, Dharana Darshan* and *Yoga Nidra* published by Yoga Publications Trust.

Research on
Asthma and Diabetes

26

Introduction

Since this book was first completed in 1977, we at the Bihar School of Yoga have gained a great deal of experience in dealing with asthma, diabetes, high blood pressure and several other supposedly incurable psychosomatic and degenerative conditions. From this experience we are convinced that yoga has a very important role to play in ultimately finding a cure for these conditions and we are correlating and conducting research to study this in greater detail.

Many people seek yogic advice for their various disease conditions and it is often surprising how easy it can be to achieve moderate to good results in a relatively short time by merely modifying the diet and introducing a little exercise and relaxation. At the same time we have found that yoga can do much more than this. It is a powerful system of manipulating our psychophysiology and, in combination with allopathy and other systems of healing, can lead to deep and complete rejuvenation of the various levels of our being. It is the ability through yoga to manipulate the internal physical and mental states via a practical and scientific system of techniques which is so important and which should be appreciated.

The yogic process is not just therapeutic for it encompasses palliation and prevention of disease and promotes health. It should be remembered that in yoga health is seen more as a side effect of the total process of mind and body integration than as an ultimate aim in itself. Ultimately good health at all levels cannot be fully attained and maintained if we do not constantly deal with all the levels of our personality in a positive manner. We must not only eliminate disease and regain our health but also ensure that we do not fall sick again, and this requires consistent effort for our whole lives. In this way we grow healthier and stronger at all levels of our being. Good health, from the yogic point of view, therefore, is seen not just as something physical and tangible that, once achieved, we can forget about, but more in the context of the ongoing process of total growth, development and evolution.

Are asthma and diabetes incurable?
The view of the medical profession is that, for the most part, asthma and diabetes are incurable conditions that we will have to learn to live with. This attitude subconsciously programs both the doctor and the patient with a defeatist, negative attitude. We hypnotize ourselves into believing that we are, and always will be sick. This may be, in itself, one of the biggest obstacles to overcoming asthma, diabetes and other psychosomatic diseases.

Yoga teaches us to change our attitude towards disease, to see it as a learning experience, and at the same time offers us the techniques by which we can not only remove disease, but also manipulate and cultivate our internal body processes so as to achieve higher states of awareness and fulfilment. In asthma, for example, it offers us techniques to relax spasmed muscles, induce bronchodilation, remove clogged mucus, rebalance the nervous system, allay anxiety and remove the root cause from the emotional and psychic body. In diabetes it lowers blood sugar and rebalances imbalanced neural and metabolic processes as well as helping us to become stronger, fitter and happier.

Chronic diseases can be the cause of untold suffering if we give in to them. However, if we see through our negativity and muster our willpower and determination, we can make the disease situation a challenge instead of a problem, and an opportunity to learn and grow. When we add yoga to our lives, it is purifying, strengthening, transformative and liberating, allowing us to make the most of our situation, whether we are asthmatic, diabetic, hypertensive or healthy.

The need for yoga

There is an obvious and pressing need for some new approach to the psychosomatic disease situation. Most asthmatics and diabetics, for example, face a progressively deteriorating situation. Ongoing illness gradually destroys the quality of their lives. It becomes increasingly difficult to participate in the normal activities of life despite the continual use of medication. Yoga claims that it is able to remedy this situation.

The need for yoga can be better appreciated when we examine the present modes of therapy available for disease situations. In asthma, for example, the situation often requires higher doses of more potent drugs more frequently. One of the most potent drugs used, cortisone, has many severe side effects and can even cause diabetes. This is a situation in which the cure may be worse than the disease itself. If yoga can, as it claims, alleviate asthma and reduce our need for potent and dangerous medicines then this, in itself, is good reason to introduce yoga into the therapeutic regime. However, yoga claims, in many cases, to do more than this and we have seen time and again that it can completely eliminate the disease. This is the author's personal experience.

In diabetes there are many doctors who state that the disease is incurable and that only insulin should be used. It is now thought that, as long as the blood sugar level can be lowered to reasonable levels, the risk of serious complications such as blindness, neuropathy, heart and kidney disease and leg ulcers, will be reduced. Certain doctors and researchers believe that only insulin can adequately control and bring down the blood sugar level, though this is contentious, and even with insulin the disease still progresses and complications usually result.

There is also evidence to support the opposite view, that too many people are being treated by insulin and there is accumulating evidence that artificial insulin may be one of the factors involved in hardening of the arteries, one of the major causes of heart attacks. Trials have shown that the need for insulin can often be reduced, if not eliminated, merely by the introduction of physical exercise and high fibre food into the diet.

Trials have also shown that yoga can reduce blood sugar levels, as well as body weight and the effects of stress and tension, factors which aggravate diabetes. If yoga can do this, then it should definitely become a part of the medical management of diabetes, especially if it can eliminate the need for insulin and oral medications which have their own bad side effects.

Yoga before complications

It is unfortunate that people often come to yoga once the disease has progressed and complications have set in. In diabetes, for example, it is an unfortunate paradox that initially the condition is relatively pain free and does not seem to be so bad to the individual concerned. There is no impetus or compulsion to look for some better method of cure, to examine the lifestyle for its weak points or to improve dietary or exercise habits. People often come to our ashram late in the disease process when it is more difficult for yoga to work.

It is for this reason that everyone should at least know about the yogic process so that if they want to, they can have the opportunity to alleviate their condition using yogic methods before complications set in. The earlier we know about yoga and apply it in our lives, the better are our chances of success. It is for this reason that doctors should advise their patients to use yogic techniques under medical guidance for the best possible management of their condition, to avoid complications and to gradually strengthen the body and mind.

Total patient health care

Most systems of healing have failed to deal adequately with psychosomatic and degenerative diseases, because they have not recognized the deeper needs of the patients at the more subtle levels of their existence. We are much more than a physical body.

According to yoga, human beings have a physical, emotional, mental, psychic and spiritual side to their existence and each level must be nourished, stimulated and developed if we are to grow into totally balanced and healthy people. It is in this regard that yoga will be most useful and helpful to modern medicine. Yoga not only outlines a clear and precise description and roadmap of the mind and our higher, more subtle aspects, but also gives us the techniques by which we can manipulate, heal, improve, cultivate and develop the mind and higher consciousness.

Most systems of healing fail to deal with the mind and fail to understand how powerful and all pervading the mind actually is. In this regard, yoga and meditative techniques are essential tools in dealing with diseases, because they cultivate and bring us into direct experience with the mind. They allow us to feel that the mind is actually enhancing and expanding our awareness. Awareness is the essence by which we can perceive more clearly how the various bits and pieces fit together, to see cause and effect, to actually feel more clearly what is going on within our own bodies, to know who we are.

We must remember that in order to treat, alleviate and eventually cure asthma and diabetes, or any psychosomatic or degenerative condition for that matter, we must deal with more than the physical symptoms. Emotional suppression or imbalance, mental anguish, anxiety and depression and psychic disturbances, must all be dealt with, and this requires a competent and experienced technician of the mind. Yoga helps us, whether we are patients, yoga teachers or doctors, to understand our own minds and, therefore, to understand the minds of others.

Yoga and medicine

Once again, it must be stated that yoga and any form of medicine work together and are not antagonistic. Allopathy, homeopathy, ayurveda, acupuncture, and other forms of healing are all useful and beneficial to mankind. They focus on and aim to eliminate the disease process. Yoga, on the other hand, is not so much therapeutic as strengthening and health-promoting, leading to good physical health, more as a by-product than as an inherent aim of the techniques. Thus, the medical tradition is required to monitor the progress of the disease and adjust drug requirements and therapeutic modes while the yogic side helps to relax, purify and strengthen, to actually aid the effects of the medicines, reduce the amounts required, and enhance tissue healing and regeneration.

Medicine and yoga work together well. If we utilize the best of both the systems, both doctor and patients must benefit. One very good way to achieve this aim of friendly cooperation and amalgamation (yoga) of the best of both worlds is for patients to visit their doctors for regular ongoing medical check-ups of their physical health. This will also allow the yoga teacher to know if the yogic methods are working. Suitable adjustments of medicines and yoga can then be made. There can no longer be any doubt that yoga is of benefit in asthma and diabetes. Doctors must retain an open mind and realize that allopathy alone actually offers very little in the psychosomatic situation, for the patient's overall well-being, for total health care. Medicines can only do so much, and they should not be the 'be-all and end-all' of medical treatment.

Yoga classes allow patients to get more time and attention for their deeper, inner personal needs, to help alleviate social, mental and emotional problems through regulated, systematic and progressive exercise and relaxation programs. The physical side benefits from this and the patient's overall condition improves.

When yoga and medicine can work together in this manner, we will be paving the way for a better world, one in which the physical, emotional, mental and deeper psychic needs of people can be catered for. This will lead to total patient health care, ultimately allowing us to transcend the present limitations of the healing professions, and endowing us with a system of attaining health, happiness and fulfilment.

27

Personal Experience

Since this book was first written, certain experiences have occurred which have, in retrospect, taught me that the root cause of asthmatic problems lies in the deeper psychic mind, within our attitudes and concepts, our self-image and attitude to people and life in general. Unless we can find effective and practical methods to affect these deeper levels of our being and thereby experience a deep change within ourselves, it is difficult, if not impossible, to eradicate our problems from our lives.

At the time of writing the original edition of this book, the yogic process was well under way. I had been learning asana, pranayama, hatha yoga shatkarma and meditation under the guidance of Swami Satyananda of the Bihar School of Yoga for some months and had experienced wonderful relief from symptoms and had been able to completely eliminate the need for any further medication.

Attacks of asthma had become less frequent and less severe and when they came they were easily managed by performing kunjal and neti, then doing Om chanting for 20 minutes and then drinking hot, black coffee. At this time I noticed that there were three important components affecting my asthma:
1. Diet
2. Allergy
3. Emotion

Diet

Diet was an important aggravating factor. Any time I ate more milk, cheese, dahi (yoghurt) or other dairy products, rice, sweets or banana than I could properly digest, I noticed that the mucus of my body would become thick and copious and exacerbated my sinusitis, allergic rhinitis, asthma and bronchitis. A heavy meal taken in the evening, especially one which was oily or fried or contained excessive dal (lentils, split peas and other pulses) caused wind and indigestion and frequently promoted an attack of asthma either before or during sleep.

Overeating was another significant predisposing factor in promoting an acute asthma attack. As I noticed this relationship, it became a meditation to discern at what point to stop eating and to try to determine which foods could be digested well and their effect upon the body and mind. Whenever food caused breathing difficulties, immediate use of kunjal (vyaghra kriya) could terminate the attack and then some form of simple pranayama or Om chanting and black coffee did the trick and brought relaxation and warmth.

Once this experience is repeated several times, it induces great self-confidence and one ceases to worry about having attacks. This new and relatively fearless attitude of mind is therapeutic in itself and each attack then becomes a challenge and an opportunity to learn how they occur, what happens during the attack and how to overcome it and thereby strengthen body and mind. At the same time we learn about our needs; for example, people suffering from asthma must always ensure not to eat more mucus-forming food than they can digest.

Allergy

Another important feature of my experience in overcoming asthma was to learn to deal with and utilize the allergic component. Whenever exposure to dust or some allergen precipitated allergic rhinitis and wheezing, the use of jala neti, saline water nasal douche, was a great help in reducing the severity of the condition, especially when cold tap water was used.

It is important in dealing with allergy through the yogic process, not to run away from the condition. We should avoid using anti-histamines as much as possible. When an attack occurs it is far preferable to use yoga and to overcome the problems gradually and systematically through our own efforts. It is, of course, difficult to appreciate this in the middle of an acute crisis and requires courage, self-discipline and experienced guidance not to resort immediately to drugs. If we wait a little while and utilize neti, pranayama, relaxation and patience, things will usually sort themselves out automatically and we will not experience the unpleasant side effects of the antihistamines.

Many times during my early stay in the ashram, I was exposed to smoke, dust, pollen and other irritants which caused sneezing or wheezing. When this occurred, I would perform the appropriate yogic practice and then resume whatever I had just been doing. Gradually, many things which would previously have caused allergic phenomena ceased to do so.

Mental attitude is an important component in the allergic side of asthma. I noticed that whenever a situation occurred which I did not like, that sneezing would start in a reflex way. Through the process of asana, pranayama and especially meditation, we can see this mental reactivity more clearly and can therefore deal with it more effectively and efficiently. If we realize the connection between mind and the disease process, it becomes a simple matter of volition, of willing ourselves to change. Whenever a situation arises in which we feel a negative mental reaction, it is important to change our attitude and to try to accept things as they are. If possible we should learn to see the good side of things, the learning possibilities, the opportunity to serve and thereby become willing to do things we previously would have rejected.

In my own case, I developed an allergy to being in contact with certain people within a certain therapeutic situation. Every time I came into that situation, though I did not realize it at the time, I developed anxiety and insecurity, fearing subconsciously, because of some traumatic past experiences, the outcome of such a meeting. For some reason then unknown to me I began to sneeze violently and could not understand why this should be so.

Later, through meditation I realized that my perception of this situation was incorrect, that there was nothing to fear and no reason for anxiety or paranoia, that the problem was in me and that if I just changed my attitude and began to enjoy the situation in a new light, as an opportunity to serve and to learn, then the external situation changed automatically for the better. Miraculously the sneezing stopped and never recurred.

Emotional release

A few months after my arrival at the Bihar School of Yoga, when everything seemed to be clearing up and I was proud of the fact that I had conquered my asthma, I was struck by a particularly severe bout of asthma and bronchitis. This attack was so severe that I could not walk about and was bedridden.

One afternoon an experience occurred that changed my life. Lying in bed and aware of all external environmental stimuli, a subconscious memory of the past arose and was so strong that I felt almost as though I were back in the past at a time certain events, narrated in the first chapter of this book, took place.

They were extremely vivid and realistic experiences. At the same time that this was taking place I realized that my whole asthma problem was arising because of an emotional paralysis, an inability to express my feelings and emotions because of an irrational fear of what others may think, the insecurity of not knowing how to handle situations and lack of self-confidence. I was unable to give of myself.

I realized that this attitude, somehow cultivated by an inability to handle and digest certain experiences from the

209

past, had caused my asthma, and had also interfered with my ability to interact with and fully live and enjoy life. At the same time I experienced a deep relaxation in the centre of my chest (anahata chakra, the heart centre) and a tremendous sense of release, relief and joy despite the physical suffering. After this, my bronchitis quickly cleared up.

Since this experience I have never again suffered from asthma or bronchitis, and I date my own cure from this time. In retrospect this was the uprooting of the psychic component of the disease, the realization that one must give of oneself, to accept and act totally without fear or anxiety. The root cause having been eliminated, the only thing remaining was to deal with the effects of the asthma on the physical, muscular and metabolic (pranic) levels.

Eliminating the last vestiges
Once the root cause of the asthma was eliminated, all that remained was to retrain the muscles and nervous system to a new, healthier mode of activity. The majority of tension and disturbance centred around the heart centre with distortion of the diaphragm and its movement, and the back muscles at the level of T4–8. This manifested as a stooping posture with compression of the chest and upper abdomen. The tension from this area was also felt to disturb the digestive process with a tendency to constipation.

Laghoo shankhaprakshalana, kunjal and neti were very effective in dealing with the residual mucus problems, alleviating spasm of the diaphragm and eliminating constipation and sinusitis. These techniques were practised often initially, even as much as daily for a month at a time. Then the frequency was reduced to once or twice per week and increased when the tendency to congestion or constipation recurred. Gradually, after 3–4 months these techniques were no longer necessary for asthma but were practised for health maintenance, prevention and the sheer joy that comes from their practice. Gradually strength and health returned and continued to grow. Eventually it was possible to leave these practices and to use them for occasional maintenance, clean-up and preventive purposes.

The postural defects were improved by the regular practice of asanas, especially surya namaskara, the asanas from shankhaprakshalana, and the major asanas listed in this book. These were instituted systematically and sequentially, to suit individual needs and according to the dictates of awareness and sensitivity to my changing physical condition.

The postures which seemed to be especially useful were: tadasana, hasta utthanasana, pada hastasana, chakrasana, paschimottanasa, bhujangasana, tiryaka bhujangasana, dhanurasana and sarvangasana. Of course, these were practised in a balanced routine with shavasana interspersed in between to aid the progressive healing effects of each practice. They worked to ease tension in the diaphragm and back, improve breathing, liberate energy in the body and develop relaxation and strength.

On one occasion when I had achieved some skill in dhanurasana for the first time, I felt a knot of energy unwind in the upper back and simultaneously and instantly my nostrils which had been blocked, inflamed and continuously dripping mucus, for many years, cleared up. The breath began to flow freely and this continued for some hours until the old condition reasserted itself. Further persistent asana practice eventually eliminated this problem completely. The whole respiratory tract became strong and well oiled.

Pranayama was especially important in overcoming diaphragmatic spasm. Nadi shodhana, bhastrika and ujjayi form the basis of the asthma program and, when combined with various mudras and bandhas, their effects are multiplied many fold.

In order to master pranayama, the full yogic breath – mastering the three stages of abdominal, thoracic and clavicular breathing – was essential. This type of breathing was alternated with pure abdominal breath awareness which allows us to see when subconscious tensions are creeping up

211

on us and causing habitual patterns of tensing in the abdominal musculature. This technique not only improves pranayama but improves breathing throughout the day as it can be practised anytime, anywhere.

In terms of breaking up diaphragmatic and muscular tension, the techniques of nauli and agnisar kriya were also very useful. Kunjal and vastra dhauti, however, remained the prime and most powerful switches to turn on and off the various components of the brain stem and autonomic nervous system.

Ultimately all the effects of hatha yoga, asana and pranayama were consolidated and improved by meditation, especially the techniques of ajapa japa, antar mouna, (witnessing, vipassana, mindfulness) and kriya yoga. These practices both uproot subconscious tensions and give us a practical means of dealing with and disposing of them. It is from these techniques that mental peace and emotional balance spring, for they enable us to develop insight and intuition concerning ourselves and our path in life.

When all these techniques are used in a balanced, systematic and progressive manner, good health and peace of mind are side effects to the attainment of fulfilment and enjoyment of life.

28

Asthma:
The Holistic Approach

Asthma is considered by many people to be an incurable disease although in children it often seems to remit spontaneously. However, even in this latter situation, the lungs remain weak and prone to disease, cough and cold, bronchitis and allergy, and the recurrence of asthma. From the yogic point of view, asthma can be easily managed so that the symptoms are lessened and the disease is completely eradicated. This is achieved by strengthening the lungs, balancing the nervous system, and uprooting the emotional tensions that are at the root of asthma. Yoga, in combination with medicine, offers us the means to achieve this.

It is our contention that asthma is a multifaceted disease which requires a multipronged approach and that many of the facets of this condition have been neglected and misunderstood accounting for the failure of traditional medical management. Once these factors are better understood and methods are devised to handle them, the asthmatic can have a better chance to escape his condition.

It is important that a better approach to management is found and anyone who has ever experienced the wheezing breathlessness of asthma can well appreciate this need. In Australia, one in 10 children and one in 20 adults are affected; between 400 and 500 people are dying each year from asthma. In America there are an estimated 10 million children suffering from asthma. The percentage of asthma

213

patients in industrially polluted towns and cities rises precipitously and in some of the coal mining and steel refining cities of India, it is one of the most common chronic disease problems that doctors and patients face.

The mechanics of asthma

One of the points least understood today is that asthma "is not just a chest disease... but is in most, if not all, cases a local manifestation in the bronchi of a generalized hyper-sensitivity, hyper-reactivity, cellular (hormonal or enzyme) imbalance... requiring biological regulation but certainly total patient care."[1] This is also the yogic and the psychosomatic view and recently the science of psychoneuro-immunology has developed to investigate the mechanisms by which the mind influences the body to trigger asthma.

Asthma can be described as paroxysmal generalized airways obstruction and is characterized by increased respon-siveness of the lungs to various factors, such as emotion, stress, allergens, cigarette smoke, exercise, respiratory tract infections, fumes, dust, alcohol, drugs such as aspirin and changes in environment and season. In the asthmatic these stimuli, which do not adversely affect normal people, cause constriction of the tubes of the lungs (bronchi), thickening of mucus and muscle spasm, resulting in wheezing and great physical and mental suffering and anguish.

In asthma there is fast, shallow respiration (increased total ventilation, hyperinflation, small tidal volume and increased frequency). Expiration is especially difficult because of collapse of the bronchi and blockage by mucus and there is a tendency to gasp for air before exhalation is completed which further compounds the problem and leads to hyperinflation. There is usually spasm of the diaphragm, making abdominal breathing difficult. Thoracic breathing with accessory muscles is used, which is a particularly inefficient system quickly leading to exhaustion.

In the lungs themselves there is disturbance of gas exchange between the lungs and the blood and lowered

214

blood oxygen levels lead to further breathlessness and weakness. Blood flow to poorly ventilated areas is also reduced. There is generalized muscle spasm in asthma and particularly diaphragmatic spasm so that only jerky movements occur. Poor posture, characterized by slouching, further reduces respiratory capacity and can also impair normal body functioning through its effect on various nervous connections.

According to Lowen and the school of bioenergy and body-personality interaction, habitual muscular tension and poor posture reflect emotional and deeper psychological tensions.[2] In the asthmatic there is a tendency to avoid expressing feelings, especially anger.[3] Asthmatics have also been found to inhibit aggression in both words and feelings, which is substituted by an abnormal pattern of respiratory behaviour.[4]

Asthma seems to exert its effect via the autonomic nervous system and via certain chemicals, such as histamine, slow reacting substance A, kinins, prostaglandins and serotonin, all of which can cause bronchoconstriction.[5] It seems more than likely that stress, emotional tension, anxiety and various psychological factors act via the central controlling centres of the brain, especially the prefrontal cortex, limbic and reticular activating systems and hypothalamic-pituitary axis. We know that stress can severely derange functioning of these structures and induce disease.[6]

Asthma is thought to result because of weakened sympathetic nervous system activity, which is probably due to ongoing stress and mental tension overactivating the sympathetic-adrenal gland system, and resulting in sympathetic-parasympathetic imbalance. There is also thought to be an imbalance in the various types of smooth muscle receptors, the alpha receptors which constrict smooth muscle in response to sympathetic activity and the beta which relax smooth muscle (e.g. in the lungs) in response to sympathetic activity; in asthma there is relative unavailability of beta receptors.

215

Summing up, the following factors are directly or indirectly involved in or are part of the asthmatic condition: disturbed respiratory function and breathing patterns, poor oxygenation of the blood, diaphragmatic and respiratory muscle spasm, generalized body muscle spasm and poor posture, emotional suppression and anxiety, and nervous system imbalance.

The holistic approach

It is obvious when we look at the factors involved in asthma that medical treatment is not adequate to deal with the emotional, mental, muscular or even the respiratory factors of asthma. The use of drugs, allergic desensitization and even physiotherapy are obviously inadequate since they are only symptomatic and palliative rather than curative.

According to Dr. John Goyeche, Associate Professor of Psychology, Department of Psychiatry, Kurume University Medical School in Japan, the poor results we are presently seeing from medical therapy "may be the result of ignoring several important psychobiological or somatopsychic characteristics, which the orthodox medical approach seems to be guilty of."[7]

He also states that, "while rather standardized procedures seemed to have evolved for the medical management of asthma, the orthodox use of steroids and bronchodilators, etc. for providing temporary relief raises a number of questions, aside from the obvious fact that many patients (and their doctors?) become psychologically dependent upon them. Both 'habituation' and 'rebound' effects are known to occur with the prolonged use of these drugs, although it appears that there has been no definitive long-term evaluation of the chronic use of these chemicals – a task which is long overdue, and which may result in some surprisingly negative conclusions about them."[8] Goyeche calls for a holistic approach to the asthma patient with much broader diagnostic measures and therapeutic range. He lists the following neglected psychosomatic factors:

216

- Most asthmatics have suppressed emotions and an inability to express emotions, especially anger and anxiety. They also suffer from excessive self-consciousness and dependency.
- This emotional suppression reflects in heightened general muscle tension which distorts posture.
- The tensions are particularly focused in chronic contraction of the voluntary muscles of respiration, and particularly in the diaphragm which becomes spasmed and jerky in its action.
- Goyeche states that, "muscle tension is probably not an outcome or aftermath of the onset of asthma, but rather is more likely a precipitating or concomitant factor: which also functions in a vicious circle fashion to perpetuate and aggravate the asthmatic syndrome."[9]
- Abnormal respiration also contributes to anxiety and the continuation of asthma in a vicious circle.

Goyeche goes on to state that a holistic therapy must be designed to deal with asthma and would have to:

- Encourage emotional release especially for aggression and sorrow.
- Teach techniques which help to release anxiety, decrease self-consciousness and increase independence and self-control.
- Teach muscle relaxation techniques.
- Teach postures or exercises to correct posture.
- Teach methods to relax irrelevant respiratory muscles to restore natural diaphragmatic breathing.
- Teach methods to expel mucus.

From our experience at the Bihar School of Yoga, this description is very close to the yogic view of the asthmatic situation and through yoga the attempt is made to tackle the total asthmatic problem almost simultaneously from all directions, giving a better chance to successfully overcome this disease.

29

Asthma:
Holistic Therapy

W hen we use an integrated, holistic yogic approach to
the treatment of asthma, we not only eradicate illness
but also gain the tools to develop control over the brain,
mind and body, thereby adding a new dimension to our
lives. Asthma then emerges as a blessing in disguise, the
awakening event which forces us to change, grow, learn and
evolve into better, more aware people.

Very few techniques or systems can meet all the
requirements for a multipronged approach to the many
facets of asthma. It is a mistake to imagine that one technique
or one drug can affect the body and mind sufficiently to
cure asthma. Even in yoga we must use several techniques
to affect muscular tension, breathing patterns and deeper
emotional, mental and neurological imbalance and tension.

In this chapter we will present several research papers
on relaxation and breathing techniques used in the treatment
of asthma. We will describe in detail how these techniques
can be incorporated in a fully integrated and balanced yogic
program to achieve one of the most systematic, comprehensive and powerful methods of eradicating asthma and
once more enjoying a healthy active life.

Relaxation

Several studies have been conducted on various forms of
relaxation and allied techniques.[1-23] Even though the results

have been encouraging and even statistically significant in several trials, few clinically significant results have emerged and several of the trials have suffered because design and analysis have been inadequate.

Erskine-Milliss and Schonell have reviewed several studies of muscular relaxation, systematic desensitization, biofeedback assisted relaxation and meditation.[24] From their study, simple muscular relaxation alone was not found to have a therapeutic role in asthma. Mental relaxation via meditation and autogenic training, and the methods of systematic desensitization were found to provide subjective and objective, clinically significant improvement. The authors state that electromyographic biofeedback is a useful adjunct to relaxation training.

According to Goyeche, relaxation and biofeedback training have shown experimental evidence for the short term reduction of asthma. However, these methods will prove to be too specific to be of any lasting value to the asthmatic on their own.[25]

This kind of research is extremely useful. However, from the practical point of view, it is better not to compare techniques on their own but rather to see how each technique can be used to help in a total and integrated system. For example, muscle relaxation training is useful before going on to mental relaxation techniques in order to break down the gross muscle tensions that prevent us from attaining deeper mental relaxation. This is the greatness of yoga – it integrates many practices and allows us to accept and utilize everything in a systematized, progressive manner, to work powerfully and simultaneously at many levels.

From the yogic point of view, relaxation training is an important supplement to the totality of yogic training; however, it is non-specific in asthma and would never be used alone. Rather, it is always used in combination with the other yogic practices. Asana, pranayama and shatkarma affect and manipulate the nervous and endocrine systems and by themselves can induce deep relaxation at physical,

219

emotional, mental and psychic levels. Relaxation techniques are used in between these techniques to help re-establish homeostasis, to allow the release of tensions, emotions and trapped energies, and to redirect these energies to work for deeper healing and regeneration of tissues and systems. It is during relaxation that the benefits gained by asana, pranayama and hatha yoga can be fully realized. Once we are relaxed, we are ready to go on to the next stage of the yogic process, which takes us a step further towards uprooting the disease from deeper emotional and psychic levels.

When we study relaxation techniques, therefore, we must view them in their correct perspective. They are not sufficient to re-establish neurological balance in asthma because the problem is more one of parasympathetic overactivity, for which we require techniques to increase sympathetic tone, the opposite of that which relaxation techniques have been shown to achieve.

At the same time there is the danger of rebound and of going too much in the opposite direction towards sympathetic overactivity. Therefore, yogis utilize techniques such as hatha yoga shatkarma, asana and pranayama, which relax peripheral muscles, dislodge mucus, aid in uprooting suppressed emotions and increase metabolic and sympathetic adrenal activity, in combination with relaxation and meditation practices. These latter techniques induce a parasympathetic dominant, hypometabolic state in which we learn to observe, witness and handle our emotional and mental tensions as they arise, in a relaxed and controlled manner. In this way we rebalance the central neurological controlling mechanisms systematically, progressively, gradually and safely and thereby regain control over our breathing mechanisms and our lives.

Retraining the breath

Physiotherapy is a medically accepted adjunct to the drug treatment of asthma. It aims to slow down and lengthen expiration so that the lungs empty fully before the next inspiration, reintroduce relaxed abdominal breathing rather than the thoracic type, reduce general muscle spasm and mobilize the ribcage and chest wall and improve postural deformity.[26] The deep breathing exercises of physiotherapy are designed to increase the lung volume, dilate airways, push air past mucus blockages and thereby aid in its expulsion during expiration, and generally retrain breathing patterns.

It is obvious that physiotherapy centres around retraining the lungs, and generally working on peripheral organs, such as muscles and ribs. This science reflects the medical view of asthma as a disease of the lungs with associated allergic and emotional components rather than the holistic view in which emotional disturbance is the prime factor triggering hypersensitivity of the lungs and immune system. This latter view is becoming more popular with the development of the science of psycho-neuro-immunology, which seeks to explain the mind-emotion-body link; however, it still has not filtered into medical consciousness and into standard medical practice or the medical textbooks. Even physiotherapy is not much accepted or used by the medical community, which relies more on drug therapeutics.

Several trials have been conducted and have demonstrated that physiotherapy can be of value in the treatment of asthma. Livingstone and Gillespie taught techniques to shorten inspiration and lengthen expiration, resembling nadi shodhana pranayama in this respect.[27] They also taught techniques involving exhaling through the mouth with a humming, whistling or hissing noise, a technique which resembles Om chanting and bhramari pranayama in this respect. Using these techniques they found that more than half of their cases became symptom free and good clinical results were obtained in 69% of cases. As asthmatics gained confidence, drugs were withdrawn and they could abort impending attacks by the exercises alone. Objective evaluation indicated increased diaphragmatic movement and improved chest expansion.

According to Barach, the humming technique reduces bronchial constriction, empties alveoli more efficiently and tends to prevent collapse of bronchi during exhalation.[28] He taught pure abdominal breathing and emphasized relaxation of abdominal musculature.

Allan taught active expiration and passive inspiration, a technique which resembles kapalbhati.[29] He found that diaphragmatic breathing increases the maximum breathing capacity and vital capacity and induces positive changes in blood count.

Erickson emphasized pulling the abdominal muscles towards the spine during exhalation, a technique which resembles both kapalbhati and bhastrika.[30]

Fein and his associates used physiotherapy and found improved chest expansion and capacity to control diaphragmatic breathing, which induced a sense of security and enabled asthmatics to abort mild attacks of asthma.[31]

A recent study at Toraman Hospital in Tokyo has shown that even emphysema benefits from diaphragmatic breathing because it allows patients to inhale more fully and reduces effort.[32] Relaxation of the abdomen and lower chest is required to perform this type of breathing.

It is an interesting observation that, even though encouraging statistical data and evidence for the effectiveness of physiotherapy has been available for several decades, doctors do not avail themselves much of its use. Perhaps it has received insufficient active propagation or perhaps facilities are lacking for its proper and easy referral.

Physiotherapy versus yoga

According to Goyeche, "While the development of the physiotherapeutic approach has served as a good corrective to drug oriented medicine, and has established the possibility of the asthmatic learning to manage himself, it can also be criticized as being too specific or 'mechanically' oriented."[33] He states that on its own, physiotherapy does not deal adequately with emotional suppression, anxiety release or muscle relaxation, and in terms of correcting posture, relaxing respiration and expelling mucus, there are better methods which are more appropriate and powerful. For this he cites yoga as being the method which best fulfils all the criteria of a holistic therapy.

Physiotherapy is a more mechanical approach than yoga, utilizing weights, belts and manual compression to aid expiration, chest tapping to loosen mucus, and postural drainage to expel mucus and to help the diaphragm ascend on expiration, utilizing gravity and the weight of the abdominal organs.

Though asana such as sarvangasana, vipareeta karani mudra, pada hastasana and pranamasana (in vajrasana) aid postural drainage, and pranayama acts to strengthen the lungs, these are more side effects of the techniques. Yoga practices are more mentally directed, though body based, and their purpose is to allow us to dive deep within ourselves so as to gain deeper awareness of who we are and what is going on within the body and mind. Thereby, again as a side effect, they confer on us the ability to actually control the central structures of the brain and therefore the mechanisms which translate emotional suppression and anxiety into endocrinal, chemical, neurological and muscular imbalance and tension and finally into bronchoconstriction.

Breath and yoga
The aim of yogic breathing techniques is to relax, balance and energize the central nervous system, and to purify the mind from subconscious tensions and suppressions. This has effects on the total body-mind complex and at the same time the lungs are strengthened as a natural result of the respiratory work performed.

Several studies have demonstrated the ability of prana-yama alone to improve lung and total body functioning. Katakov reports that the use of ujjayi at the rate of one breath per minute increases breath holding capacity and decreases breath volume, oxygen uptake and release of carbon dioxide.[34] This indicates a hypometabolic state and the capacity for pranayama to affect and adjust the regulating mechanisms in the brain.

Tengshe has found that pranayama such as ujjayi, bhastrika and kapalbhati, influence respiratory, cardiovascular, metabolic and neural functions, with increased EEG synchronization accompanied by a subjective attitude of mental quietude and alert restfulness; a relaxed, internally aware state.[35] He states that these practices influence the basic profile of various body functions (and this probably acts via central brain controls) "indicating an overall improvement in respiratory functions, in physical efficiency and subjective feeling of general well-being, a tendency towards parasympatheticotonic type cardiovascular reactivity, and reduction in free fatty acid level in the blood probably suggesting reduction in catecholamine and sympathetic activity."

Pranayama is usually preceded by asana, dynamic movements or static postures, which themselves utilize slow, controlled breathing and the development of awareness. Certain postures such as the inverted asana, sirshasana and sarvagasana, and the forward bending paschimottanasana and shashankasana, facilitate exhalation because of the weight of abdominal contents on the diaphragm and/or compression of the chest. Backward bending asana facilitate inhalation because of natural expansion of the chest by the posture. Certain twisting postures facilitate unilateral expansion of one side of the chest and concomitant compression of the other side.

In the asthma situation asana in combination with pranayama help to increase the movement of the diaphragm, increase vital capacity, increase inspiration and expiration duration and increase expulsion of mucus. This latter is probably maximal in inversion. Asana probably also act to improve the perfusion of oxygen into the blood and certainly the exercise component of asana improves cellular respiration and makes oxygen utilization more efficient.

224

It should be remembered that the aim of asana and pranayama is not to improve breathing, though this occurs anyway. Rather, they are designed to influence the entire postural regulating mechanism in the brain and to learn higher conscious control over subconscious autonomic processes. At the same time we develop deep muscular and visceral relaxation, physical health, steadiness of body and mind, stamina, and the ability to enter higher states of meditation. As we become more aware of these deep primitive circuits and reflexes and gain control over them, energy can be redirected to higher neural circuits to awaken latent capabilities and higher awareness.

According to Kuvalyananda and Vinekar, yoga asana affect the 'intrinsic postural substrate' through the tonic-interoceptive system, primarily by means of disinhibiting the inhibitory control of the cortex over automatic, subconscious brain stem function.[36]

Pranayama is the stage prior to meditation in which a wakeful, internal state is achieved that is initially hypometabolic and parasympathetic dominant. Pranayama is therefore much more than just breathing exercises and physiotherapy. Rather it is part of a total system of reintegration, rebalancing and reharmonizing of the body and mind, a system that purifies and strengthens, thereby eliminating tension and weakness from the body and mind. At the same time these practices awaken the inner awareness.

Controlling the brain

It is a very limited and naive view to think of yoga and pranayama purely as a means to improve lung function and oxygenation of the blood. These things do happen; however, yoga provides techniques to both increase and decrease oxygen uptake depending on their relaxing or stimulating nature and the needs of the individual in terms of attaining balance. Indeed, one of the main aims of pranayama practice is eventually to increase carbon dioxide in the body, not oxygen.

Carbon dioxide level is one of the most potent stimulators of the brain's respiration controlling centres and inspiration and expiration is continually adjusted to maintain this chemical balance in the body. Even a small increase of blood carbon dioxide will stimulate the brain to increase respiration in order to increase its elimination.

The aim of most pranayama, kumbhaka (breath retention), bandha (locks) and meditation practices is gradually, over a long period of time, to slow respiration and increase the capacity to withstand and endure carbon dioxide retention. If we can do this, it strengthens the capacity to control other facets of the brain and mind and also maintain nervous system stability and internal wakefulness during higher states of meditation.

Schulte and Abhyankar state, "Yogic breathing produces gradual accumulation of carbon dioxide which stimulates the cerebral circulation and engenders mental tranquillity and the reduction of sympathetic activity in the autonomic nervous system."[37]

Stanescu and his associates showed that the use of ujjayi, at the rate of one breath per minute, not only decreased ventilation and rate of breathing and increased tidal volume and end tidal carbon dioxide pressures, but also significantly decreased the individual's responsiveness to carbon dioxide in comparison to controls.[38] The authors state that this is due to yoga's capacity to affect the breathing control mechanism (bulbopontine pacemaker) in the brain. On the basis of their finding, they state that, "Voluntary control of breathing may be a useful adjunct in the treatment of patients with chronic obstructive lung disease and bronchial asthma."

Miles has shown that 20 minutes of ujjayi pranayama raised oxygen consumption merely 12–15% above basal needs.[39] This should be compared with the 230% increase in consumption which occurs when we move from sitting still to level walking at two miles per hour, a very gentle, undemanding pace. Pratap states that respiratory training, consciously and persistently overriding the usual stimuli from the brain's respiratory centres, "may serve to fortify an individual against the early onset of hypoxia (low oxygen levels) in emergencies concerned with oxygen supply."

In terms of the respiratory system, these and other studies indicate that asana, pranayama and meditation confer upon us control of the medulla oblongata and pons in the brainstem and the higher more conscious levels, for example, in the hypothalamus via the cortical centres.

By controlling the breath we can control our reactions to emotion and anxiety until such a time as we master the mind through meditation, when the normal stresses and strains of life can no longer affect us negatively. This is the ultimate psychotherapy for the asthmatic patient. Pratap suggests that pranayama acts via the vagus nerve and the pontive apneustic centres in the brain. This somehow alters the ascending reticular activating system to suppress sensory input to the cortex and thereby brings about steadiness of mind.[40]

Schulte and Abhyankar report the case of a 16 year old asthmatic boy who had been treated with a maintenance dose of aminophylline and cortisone since the age of 8 years, with occasional hospitalizations.[41] Using asana and pranayama he was able to reduce his medication so that he only resorted to it when necessary and felt significant improvement. The authors state that, "Since he was able to cope with anxiety without asthma attacks, his self-esteem increased considerably."

In terms of yoga's ability to control the brain, one of the most important pieces of research has recently come from the Salk Institute for Biological Sciences in California.[42] David Shannahoff-Khalsa has shown that there is a direct relationship between brain activity and the nasal cycle of alternation of congestion and decongestion in the nasal passages. They showed that when airflow is free in one nostril the opposite hemisphere is currently dominant. Forceful breathing through the more congested nostril awakens the less dominant hemisphere.

This research shows us that yogis utilized the nose and breath as a means of altering brain activity. The whole science of pranayama and swara yoga is based on this. This discovery extends the functions of the nose far beyond merely being an apparatus for smell. This research also tends to prove the contention that yogic breathing and meditation techniques are the doorways to control of the total nervous, endocrine and immune system and the whole metabolism of the body. Shannahoff-Khalsa states that this finding has major implications for developing techniques of self-regulation and shows that we can "non-invasively, selectively and predictably alter cerebral activity and associated physiologic processes."[43]

The implications of this research for asthma and other psychosomatic diseases are enormous.

Summing up

Based on our own research and experience and according to the experience of others, it is our view that drugs are not essential in the initial treatment of asthma and indeed should not be used until it is absolutely essential. This is, of course, provided the asthmatic patient has some substitute therapy, such as yoga and physiotherapy or anything that works for them, by which muscle spasm and bronchoconstriction can be reduced.

If these methods do not work, then medicines can be used. However, with time and perseverance and a little practice and experience, the attacks become less frequent and severe and it becomes easier and easier to handle and overcome asthma. Of course, this is not always possible and it is often difficult to restrain oneself so as not to jump up immediately and grab for medicines. This applies to both patient and doctor, and occurs when we panic because fear envelops the mind and forces us to act.

To overcome this natural tendency requires a higher degree of maturity, self-confidence and training in a system which offers relaxation and improved breathing. This can

228

be achieved, for example, after some weeks of yoga training which incorporates exercises, breathing techniques and relaxation – a balanced approach to both body and mind.

Education of the patient by the doctor is also necessary for it is every patient's right to know that if they follow only the drug line, they will most probably require medicines for their whole lives. They should also know that drugs such as cortisone can cause diabetes and other serious problems that may be worse than the asthma itself. We have, for example, experienced the situation in which an individual has been able to overcome asthma through yoga but has had great difficulty in stopping steroid medications.

Once patients are aware of the serious side effects and drawbacks of medication they are much more motivated to do something constructive about their health. When we experience the beneficial effects and the joy of practising yoga, it becomes an essential component of our lives; good health and happiness are natural consequences.

30

Diabetes Research

The first written record of diabetes was discovered on an ancient Egyptian papyrus dated back to 1500 BC, which described excessive urination, polyuria, one of the main symptoms of diabetes. The Indian text *Susruta*, written in approximately 400 BC, notes the disease and calls it *madhu meh*, honey in the urine. In the West, Willis first noticed the disease was characterized by sweetness of the urine in 1675. Today there are an estimated 300 million cases of diabetes in the world with possibly an equal number of undetected, symptom-free diabetics. In India it is estimated that approximately 2% of the population, 15 million people, have diabetes. In the USA there are an estimated 5 million people being treated for diabetes and another 5 million are expected to develop it sometime in their lives. The number of cases is said to be rising by 6% each year.

The disease is not just a case of having too much sugar in the blood; it affects nearly every organ in the body. An estimated 300,000 people die from diabetes and its complications such as heart attack, stroke and kidney failure. It is also the leading cause of blindness in America, as well as causing high blood pressure, impotence, gangrene and chronic infections, which often necessitate amputation. After cancer and heart disease, diabetes is the third most common cause of death in America. The American Diabetes Association has used a poster requesting funds for research with the slogan: "Every 60 seconds another American is diagnosed as diabetic."

Cause unknown

Since 1921 the discovery of insulin has saved millions of lives. However, even though the disease is one of the earliest recorded in history and despite the fact that hundreds of millions of dollars are being poured into its research all over the world, it is still poorly understood and remains the cause of untold suffering, disability and premature mortality.

Since the early pioneering work of Minkowski and the classical studies of Banting and Best, the intimate relationship between the secretion of insulin from the pancreas and clinical diabetes mellitus has been well established. However, insulin deficiency is not always the primary factor responsible for diabetes. Today there is a good deal of contention as to the exact mechanism involved. For example, some people have found altered tissue responsiveness to a normal amount of blood insulin, circulating insulin antagonists (chemicals which act against insulin), abnormalities in insulin binding and abnormalities in the insulin, glucagon ratios. There is probably some truth in all these factors.

It appears, therefore, that in diabetes one of two things can happen: either we run out of insulin, now called type 1 insulin dependent diabetes, or something goes wrong with the insulin glucose metabolism so that insulin is available but comes too late and does not work properly. This is called type 2 diabetes, not dependent on insulin.

The diabetes situation is complicated and difficult to research because sugar metabolism is so basic, all-pervasive, essential and complex. We do know that poor diet, sedentary lifestyle, obesity and mental tension are related factors, but what really goes on and how to cure it is still unknown.

Glucose metabolism

Apart from oxygen, glucose is the most important energy source in the body and is required to maintain the life and proper functioning of every cell in the body. When we eat glucose, it is transported to all the various tissues of the body as fuel and also is stored for later use. The liver, pancreas and adrenal glands are the main body organs responsible for regulating sugar metabolism.

Storage of glucose and entry of glucose into the cells of the body requires insulin. When glucose enters the body, it triggers the release of insulin from the beta cells of the islets of Langerhans in the pancreas. Insulin opens the door for glucose to enter the liver, fat and muscle cells, where it will be stored and used. Storage, the job of the liver and fat cells, is important because glucose is our most precious fuel, without which the brain and body cannot function. However, if we run out of insulin, no matter how much sugar we have available in the bloodstream, it is useless because there is no insulin to push glucose into the cells where it is needed.

Glucagon is a hormone that is released from the alpha cells of the islets of Langerhans and works opposite to insulin. It is released in response to starvation, severe exercise and carbohydrate restriction, so as to release stored glucose.

When we fast, about four or more hours after eating, insulin levels decrease and the liver automatically releases glucose to feed the body. Stress, increased sympathetic nervous system activity and adrenal gland activity, release more glucose into the blood. When we are tense, tired, under some kind of real or imagined threat or doing physical exercise, the sympathetic and adrenal systems release glucose to feed the overactive cells in the body.

The whole question of glucose metabolism is complex, multifactorial and interrelated with the workings of the whole body. It is an extremely complicated process but this provides a broad and general outline of how things work.

The psychological side

Despite the fact that in the seventeenth century, Willis himself stated that psychological factors such as 'prolonged sorrow' can be the cause of diabetes, this side of the problem is probably the least well understood. Although we know that diabetes is related to a lack of insulin, caused either by its non production or reduced production, or by its decreased or mistimed secretion, the original cause may not be in the pancreas at all.

Pancreatic secretions are controlled by the autonomic nervous system. Balance between the parasympathetic and sympathetic components is required for total body health as well as for blood sugar metabolism. We know that emotional and mental disturbance create autonomic nervous system, endocrine gland and metabolic imbalance via the limbic system in the brain, and this appears to be a major factor in diabetes, especially the maturity onset form. Stress and tension cause increased activity of the sympathetic nervous system and adrenal glands, which inhibits insulin secretion. Ongoing stress and tension are, therefore, important factors in diabetes.

It is well known that even in young children, diabetes can be precipitated by the stress of an infection, the psychic trauma of a school examination, or a fight with a friend. Only 11% of children with juvenile diabetes have a parent who also suffers from the disease. Inherited factors are, therefore, not so important in juvenile diabetes. In maturity onset diabetes, however, there are an estimated 85% of cases in which a parent is also diabetic. Strangely enough, it is the maturity onset diabetic who responds more easily to yoga practices. This may indicate that though genetic factors underlie diabetes and predispose us to weakness in certain areas, these are not the dominant determining factors. Genetics can, in most cases, be overridden by correct lifestyle, correct thinking and yoga practices.

Harris has demonstrated the importance of relaxation training in diabetes.[1] Twelve people with diabetes were randomly allocated either to a relaxation training group or to a control group which read about diabetes. Nine people completed the seven day program which consisted of three one-hour clinic sessions and four home practice sessions.

Psychological and physiological parameters were taken on each day of the test and then followed up for the following four weeks. It was found that the diabetics tended to have higher than normal anxiety in each of the five situation subscales of the S–L inventory of general trait anxiety. Some of the subjects were able to predict their physiological state from subjective cues, and a strong relationship between diabetic control and anxiety was seen. Though relaxation training decreased anxiety more than reading, the time period of the program was insufficient to reduce anxiety.

This trial points out that anxiety is an important component of the diabetic syndrome, though its role is still to be determined. Relaxation therapy has always been an important part of the yogic management of diabetes and we have constantly noticed that people coming for diabetic management have had concomitant anxiety or depression plus various stress related disorders. Reduction of tension and sympathetic overactivity is an important initial phase of training and is essential to lead into the asana, pranayama and hatha yoga shatkarma which are, from our experience, the more important techniques to drop blood sugar. However, the yogic approach requires a balance, a synthesis of activity and relaxation for best results. Activity releases tension and stimulates energy while the relaxation allows regeneration to take place.

Exercise

Celsus first advocated exercise as a component of diabetes management around the time of Christ.[2] In the 1970s, Fred Whitehouse, past president of the American Diabetes Association, stated that, "Exercise is being rediscovered as an important modality of treatment in diabetes by scientists who now need to identify how it works."[3] Philip Felig, professor of medicine and chief of endocrinology at the Yale University School of Medicine, New Haven, Connecticut, has found that exercise improves the absorption of glucose.[4] His study shows that insulin mediated blood glucose

234

uptake increased by 30% after training, in direct proportion to the increase in maximal aerobic capacity.

Greg Peterson, at the University of California in San Francisco School of Medicine, showed that after exercise, platelet stickiness dropped from 74–53% in diabetics and from 40–36% in normal subjects.[5] Platelet stickiness is thought to predispose us to blood clots and arterial disease, one of the major causes of complications, such as blindness (retinopathy) in diabetes.

It is important to remember, however, that while asana give us the benefit of exercise, they are much more than this and act to improve physical fitness as well as inducing relaxation. They can also affect our metabolism, nervous system and endocrine glands in ways that exercise cannot. Pokordi and his associates have shown that after muscular exercise, there was an increase in lactic acid in the blood and the level came down ten minutes after exercise finished.[6] In asana however, there was a drop in the level of lactic acid. After six months of regular practice, the normal resting level of lactic acid in those doing muscular exercise was high, while in those doing asana and meditation it was lowered.

Pokordi and his associates also found decreased levels of vanillyl mandelic acid (VMA), MHPG and homovanillic acid (HVA) after six months of asana and meditation, whereas in muscular exercise VMA was high but MHPG and HVA levels were not affected. There was also an accentuation of alpha and beta brain waves in those people practising asana and meditation but no such changes in people practising exercises. This indicates that the yoga practices can affect us at levels which normal exercise and physiotherapy cannot.

Correct practice is essential
Often people come to learn yoga specifically for diabetes, having practised asanas alone for many years, and are surprised that they have developed diabetes. Others have learned some asanas and pranayama practices for diabetes,

235

but have not been able to rid themselves of the disease. These people generally ask, "If we have been practising yoga, why are we sick?" The reasons are as follows:

1. Usually people are irregular in yoga practice. Regularity and perseverance are the most important keys to success.
2. They do not perform their practices correctly, performing them more as physical exercises and usually straining themselves, rather than doing the practices slowly, with correct breath synchronization and awareness. Hurry and strain in asana or pranayama can weaken the body and predispose it to many disorders, even hypertension and diabetes. The practices must be slow and relaxed and followed by shavasana to allow body homeostasis and balance to reassert itself.
3. Their practice program is insufficient, for example, they do not practise either hatha yoga or meditation.

Some form of simple meditation is essential in the uprooting of deeper psychic problems and tensions which form the core and basis of many disease entities. Unless we uproot, affect or modify these habitual, reactive patterns of thinking, emotion and behaviour, it is unlikely that we will be able to eliminate the disease process from our lives. Of course, meditation also has profound physiological effects on the brain and limbic system, and therefore on the total controlling mechanism of the body via the automatic nervous system and endocrine glands. It is more than likely that it also beneficially affects the immune system.

Shankhaprakshalana

In the treatment of diabetes, it is the practice of shankha-prakshalana that seems to make all the difference. In our own clinical trials with diabetes, we have noticed that blood sugar levels are only minimally affected in the first stages of learning asana and pranayama. However, as soon as laghoo shankhaprakshalana is instituted, dramatic falls in blood sugar levels have been recorded. It is important to remember this when teaching yoga to diabetics in order to reduce or stop insulin intake during the period in which laghoo shankhaprakshalana is being learned. Once this is done and adequate blood tests performed, we can reinstate insulin as required, though often, especially in maturity onset diabetes, this is not necessary.

Shankhaprakshalana is a much more powerful technique than its short form, laghoo shankhaprakshalana, because it completely strips the intestinal tract of food, mucus, waste products and intestinal secretions. This may require 20–30 glasses of warm, salty water while laghoo requires only 4–8 glasses of water. However, laghoo's effect is remarkably powerful and, in fact, we have found that in most cases it is sufficient to drop blood sugar levels in the majority of maturity onset, non-insulin dependent, type 2 diabetics.

Both shankhaprakshalana and its short form of laghoo induce remarkable degrees of physical and mental purification and relaxation. It is very common for people to comment after these practices on how light and relaxed they feel, both physically and mentally, tangibly experiencing the somopsychic links. How this works is a matter of conjecture, however, the following hypotheses may account for this:

1. Local cleansing and purification of the digestive tract improves the digestive process and affects and strengthens the whole body. H.S. Shukla and his colleagues compared normal preoperative bowel preparation, which involves dietary restrictions, laxatives, antibodies and enema, with total gut irrigation, TGI, a modified form of shankhaprakshalana.[7] In this technique the whole gut is flushed from mouth to anus, using 0.9% saline water on the night before operation. Shukla found that the TGI group had less post-operative infection, less wound breakdown, and less time in hospital, than the control group. The TGI group reported no post-operative deaths while in the control group one person died from infection. The surgeons themselves were, on the whole, more satisfied with the TGI.

237

2. The passage of warm, saline water through the digestive tract creates osmotic pressure which may suck out various waste products and speed up the process of elimination which is often sluggish and constipated. The process may be likened to that of dialysis.

3. Cleansing the mucous membranes with salt water is soothing and healing in itself. It often occurs that subclinical inflammation of the digestive mucosa occurs, perhaps due to impacted faeces and mucus, or parasitic infestation, or some minor inflammatory process may occur due to an ingested allergen or even an auto-immune process. These foci of inflammation create subconscious discomfort and may even initiate a kind of loop circuit of irritation in the nervous system which eventually builds up into a clinical picture. This has been found, in our experience, to be a possible cause of allergy, epilepsy, various digestive disorders and generalized debility. Warm, saline water cleans and soothes inflammation and gently stimulates the nervous system via the autonomic nervous system. We have also found that shankha-prakshalana tends to induce parasympathetic dominance and even drowsiness so that the vicious circle of spasm of sympathetic activity and disease is broken and a more relaxed state instituted in its place. This process tends to bring about a reduction in the blood sugar levels.

4. Repeated cleansing of the mucous membranes of the intestines may have a reflex action on the cell membranes of other body tissues via the various channels of tissue and cellular communication and thereby tend to improve the action of insulin on the cell membranes. The effects at the chemical and molecular levels are extremely difficult to ascertain, but we can assume that there must be some effect and that it will be benevolent if we feel better after the practice.

5. The yogi must manipulate the body via asana in order to perform the practices and push the warm, salty water through the intestinal sphincters. This forces him to

learn how to control the inner organs and thereby brings the more subtle and autonomic components of the nervous system under conscious control. This aids rebalance and reintegration of the controlling brain structures.

6. Internal stimulation of the various internal cavities and linings of the body stimulates and brings previously subconscious areas of the body into the field of conscious awareness. The process is intensified when shatkarma are practised in combination with asana, pranayama and meditation practices. This has a dual effect. It brings about awareness of the internal state of being. We can actually feel more clearly what is going on inside the body. This results in an automatic change in lifestyle, eating habits, exercise patterns and mental state, because increased sensitivity automatically prevents us from abusing the body as we may previously have done when we were less aware. Awareness prevents us from hurting ourselves in our ignorance.

Awareness has its own intrinsic rewards. Knowledge of our inner state, needs and desires, capacities and limitations leads to autonomy, self-reliance, independence and self-confidence, which are very important in dealing with the disease situation. It is also a yogic dictum that awareness of a certain part of the body automatically brings energy and rejuvenation to that part because there is a natural tendency to relaxation and rebalance.

Integrated sadhana

All yogic techniques have beneficial effects which compound themselves when practised in conjunction with each other and in a correctly balanced sadhana program. In the long term, no practice is more important than any other for each helps the other and leads on systematically and progressively to better and healthier states of being. In yogic terms the shatkarma cleanse and purify; the asana open the nadi flows of energy; pranayama circulates energy; and meditation purifies, strengthens and reintegrates the mind, ultimately leading to higher states of awareness.

No matter which physiological process is eventually proven to be responsible for the wonderful relaxation and well-being afforded by yogic practice, we can always look to the yogic texts which revered these teachings in almost sacred terms. For these were techniques which can remove disease and endow the body with strength and a vitality which makes us shine with the joy of living.

31

Case Histories

Case History 1

Mr Ashis K. Srivastava, aged 53, chief architect and city planner for Bokaro Steel City, arrived in Munger in August 1983, complaining of diabetes mellitus since 1972. His father was diabetic. His own diabetes was so bad that it required 40–50 units of insulin per day for control. Diet and oral medication had proved inadequate. He attributed much of his problem to the tremendous stress he was under at work, irregularity of meals, and the other usual problems associated with a high pressure work situation.

He arrived at Bihar School of Yoga on 15th August and was advised to stop his medications and began to learn a few simple asana and pranayama. On the 17th August blood sugar levels were taken, fasting 182 mg/100 mls and postprandial 286 mg/100 mls. He then restarted insulin at 40 units. On August 19th he practised laghoo shankha-prakshalana, kunjal and neti and was advised to halve his insulin intake. Even at this dosage he suffered a mild hypoglycaemic attack which forced him to ingest glucose. He then stopped his insulin intake. On the 23rd August his postprandial blood sugar level was 112 mg/100 mls and remained at normal levels at least until June 1984, the last date recorded.

In yogic management it is quite common to see a rapid drop in blood sugar in maturity onset diabetics on oral

241

medication. It is more rare in insulin dependent diabetes in our experience. Mr Srivastava states, "Both my wife and I are carrying on the yoga practices in the morning but on account of my heavy work load, which often keeps me glued in my office until almost 7:30 p.m., I have not been able to do pranayama or meditation at night. However, what I am able to do in the morning, is giving me much benefit both physically and psychologically, and I feel so grateful to the Bihar School of Yoga for giving this exposure for living life with all its fullness." (June 4, 1984)

When we see case histories like this and the experiences of the many people who come to the Bihar School of Yoga, it is difficult for us to believe the doctors who tell us that diabetes mellitus is incurable.

Case history 2

This case history is another example of the efficacy of laghoo shankhaprakshalana in the therapeutic situation. A 43 year old gentleman came to the ashram in March 1982 complaining of an 8 year history of diabetes. He had a fasting blood sugar level of 200 mg%, and this had been brought down by dietary control plus 3 tablets of 'daonil' per day to a fasting level of 120 mg%.

This gentleman was depressed, lethargic and yogically diagnosed as having manipura chakra debility. A course of simple practices – pawanmuktasana parts 1 and 2, surya namaskara, yogic breathing, nadi shodhana, shavasana, laghoo shankhaprakshalana, kunjal and neti – was prescribed.

After some days of asana and pranayama, laghoo shankhaprakshalana was attempted successfully. At this point in the treatment, both patient and therapist noticed a definite change. The patient was obviously brighter, happier and exhibited less psychomotor retardation. Although he found laghoo shankhaprakshalana difficult, he felt that the effects were so encouraging that it was worth the effort.

He was advised to continue asana and pranayama daily, laghoo shankhaprakshalana and kunjal daily for one month, alternate days for the month, twice weekly for one month and then once per week.

One month after commencing the practices, he stopped all his medication. He had reduced his dosage gradually over one month. Fasting blood sugar level one week after stopping medications was 92%. He has continued his sadhana.

A few months later we received a letter from his brother enquiring about yoga therapy for himself. He stated that his brother had changed so much for the better that it was difficult to imagine that he had ever been sick in his life. Even his wife had trouble readjusting to his new level of energy and vitality.

32

Yoga Therapy Camps

Between September 1982 and June 1984, the Bihar
School of Yoga conducted several health management
camps for asthma, diabetes and blood pressure. These were
held at Kanpur (U.P.), Jamshedpur (Bihar), Bhagalpur
(Bihar) and Begusarai (Bihar), in conjunction with various
groups of medical professionals.

Aim of the camps
All of these camps were aimed to be therapeutic events.
They were not designed to be controlled, clinical trials but
rather were preliminary trials from which further therapeutic research work could be designed. It was felt that
before more detailed and controlled research could be carried
out, such trials would be useful to point out the possible
traps, pitfalls and weaknesses in a research program,
particularly within the Indian context. They were also
designed to demonstrate to the medical community that
yoga is able to beneficially affect disease and that it is a
useful therapeutic regime.

ASTHMA AND DIABETES CAMP, KANPUR

The diabetes and asthma camp held at Kanpur in September
1982 was a highly successful event at both the clinical and
research levels. All the diabetic patients who completed the

244

course were found to have significantly lowered their blood sugar levels after stopping their medicines.

The G.S.V.M. Medical College, Kanpur (U.P.), extended close cooperation and took readings for both asthmatics and diabetics.

Diabetes research

Thirty patients presented themselves as being diabetic, and after screening, 14 patients were found to have a positive diabetic history. Of these 14 patients, 3 did not complete the course.

Ages ranged from 33–56 years. All were maturity onset diabetics and 9 were taking medication at the time the camp started. Of these 9 people, 4 still showed elevated blood sugar levels.

At the start of the course all patients stopped their medications and continued their diabetic diet. Fasting and postprandial (1–2 hours after food) blood sugar levels were taken. They then began a course which covered the following practices:

1. *Asana:* Pawanmuktasana 1 and 2, surya namaskara, shashankasana, ushtrasana and vajrasana.
2. *Pranayama*: Nadi shodhana, bhramari and ujjayi.
3. *Hatha yoga shatkarma*: Laghoo shankhaprakshalana, kunjal and neti.
4. *Relaxation*: Yoga nidra and simple ajapa japa.

At the end of the two week course, fasting and postprandial blood sugar levels were taken again. All the subjects expressed their feeling of subjective well-being and freedom from such symptoms as tension, headaches and digestive ailments, after the course.

Results

The following table describes the results of the trial. (F = fasting, PP = postprandial; all values are in milligrams percent (mg%). Normal F is equal to 80–120; normal PP is equal to less than 140 (mg%).

245

Patient	11.9.1982		20.9.1982	
1	F 80	PP155	F80	PP120
2	F105	PP175	F80	PP140
3	F 80	PP100	F85	PP135
4	F 85	PP140	F75	PP125
5	F 95	PP190	F80	PP135
6	F 80	PP190	F90	PP155
7	F 75	PP120	F85	PP130
8	F150	PP250	F96	PP130
9	F 95	PP180	F90	PP140
10	F124	PP168	F	PP116
11	F 80	PP150	F78	PP125

It should be noted that the blood levels on September 11, 1982 were taken 2–3 days after stopping diabetic medication which may have still been exerting an effect, even though it was wearing off. This may explain the apparently normal first blood values for patients 3, 4 and 7. It is also probable, in terms of patient compliance and understanding, that some of these people may have taken medication even after being told to stop. After reinforcement of the instructions, all patients eventually stopped medications, so that the second blood values are an accurate indication of blood sugar minus the effects of medication.

Patients 1, 2, 5, 6, 8, 9, 10 and 11 obviously show diabetes or a diabetic tendency before starting yoga. Patient 1 was a known diabetic for 15 years, taking medications on a daily basis. Patient 2 recorded F270 on the 23.8.79 and was not adequately controlled by medications. Patient 3 recorded F125, PP180 on 3.8.75 and was also controlled by medication. Patient 4 recorded F100, PP200 on 17.9.78 and was controlled by medications. Patient 5 recorded F172 on the 8.9.82 and PP231 on the 7.9.82. Patient 6 recorded PP252 on 7.9.82. Patient 7 could not locate his old medical records; however, he stated that he was definitely a diabetic and was currently taking diabetic medication. Patient 11 had a past history of PP185.

Discussion on diabetes

It became obvious to us that future camps and research will require better selection and preparation of patients. Medications should be stopped at least one week before starting yoga and blood sugar levels should be recorded then. A better plan for assessing the effects of individual practices will have to be worked out.

Long-term follow-up of the cases was to have taken place, but lack of patient compliance caused this side of the project to be abandoned.

This research as it stands highlights two very important points valuable from both the patient's and the doctor's point of view. The first is that yoga has been able to dramatically lower blood sugar levels quickly and effectively, without the need of medicines and therefore minus the risk of side effects. The second point is that all the patients experienced subjective well-being.

Asthma research

At the Kanpur camp 18 people showed a definite past history of asthma, and of these 14 completed the two-week course. Their ages ranged from 14–70 years and their asthma ranged from mild seasonal attacks to severe, chronic, obstructive airways disease. Of the 14, 10 were randomly selected for lung function measurement at the G.S.V.M. Medical College.

Out of the 10 subjects, 8 had completed the tests by the end of the two-week period. The tests included vital capacity (VC), forced expiratory volume (FEV), and haemoglobin (Hb).

Results

The 8 patients who completed the tests were divided into 2 groups: those taking steroids on a regular basis or requiring steroids for their acute attacks, and those who did not require steroids. Group 1, steroid dependent asthmatics, comprised 6 patients who all showed worsening or no improvement of their FEV, and of these only 1 improved the VC. This group of subjects had been taking steroids for a period of time ranging from 1–27 years. The subject who improved the VC had been taking steroids only when suffering from acute asthma. Group 2, the remaining 2 participants who had not taken steroids, had shown considerable improvement of FEV, but not of VC, which actually decreased in one patient.

Discussion on asthma

In the yogic treatment of asthma, subjective improvement is usually seen after two weeks, though improvement may take up to six months of therapy depending on the degree of severity of the disease. The non-steroid group, being the least severe, showed improvement after two weeks while the steroid group fluctuated from remission to exacerbation. The subjects who did not take steroids, apart from the rapid improvements in FEV, also remarked that they experienced a marked degree of subjective benefit. FEV is an important test in the evaluation of asthma because it measures the ease of expiration and asthma is a disease in which expiration is impaired.

The subjects who took steroids were advised to halve the dose of their medication at the midpoint of the yoga course. After a few days, they experienced difficulty in breathing, especially at night. This is most probably due to the fact that steroids, being extremely potent drugs, had suppressed adrenal function, and when the drugs were reduced, imbalance was created in the body's homeostatic mechanisms. It is interesting that, despite the fact that the patients were not taking their normal dose of drugs and were experiencing difficulty in breathing, they could manage to cope with their difficulty through yoga and did not have to resort back to the full dose of steroids. We interpreted this as meaning that

248

they were, in effect, starting to gain freedom from the need to use steroids, which is in itself a very difficult step towards a cure.

It is interesting to note that so many of the asthmatics were taking steroids even at a young age. Steroids are the last resort in the chemotherapeutic approach to asthma. They should not be taken unless it is absolutely necessary. Once the asthmatic starts on this course on a regular basis, it is very difficult to stop. By supplying an external source of steroids we suppress the body's own production, and may become dependent on these tablets with all their possibly dangerous side effects (e.g. diabetes), which are extremely distressing and possibly create worse conditions than the asthma itself.

Yoga therapy works on the premise that the hatha yoga shatkarma, asana, pranayama and relaxation and other practices, can stimulate the balanced production of steroids and hormones within the body as well as rebalancing the autonomic nervous system via its effect on the central controlling structures of the brain. This is absolutely preferable to the use of potent and dangerous medicines. We feel that doctors owe it to their patients to allow them a trial run of yogic techniques before resorting to the more potent medicines available. Patients should be aware of the dangers of medicines and request from their doctors the chance to use only simple drugs plus yoga before stronger drugs are used.

All the subjects taking steroids in our trial program said that these medicines gave only temporary relief and, as time went on, they required higher dosages. Their lives were still felt to be miserable. All experienced temporary relief from yoga and stated that they felt this relief immediately after the practices were completed in the morning and that it seemed easier to go without their drugs. Most were keen to give yogic therapy a trial over six months and to use steroids and other medicines only when absolutely necessary.

ASTHMA, DIABETES AND HYPERTENSION CAMP, JAMSHEDPUR

A yoga camp was held in Jamshedpur (Bihar) from 30th January to 8th February 1983 for patients with asthma, diabetes and blood pressure. More than 100 people participated in the course which was held over 10 days. They were taught asana, pranayama, meditation, relaxation and hatha yoga shatkarmas. The medical parameters were recorded with the cooperation of TISCO, TATA Main Hospital, M.G.M. Medical College and the Blood Bank.

Diabetes research

Six patients with diabetes were measured before and after yoga for fasting, postprandial and urine sugars. Oral medicines were stopped a few days before the camp began; however, it is possible that the effects of the medicines were still being experienced and that the 'before' readings were slightly inaccurate on this account. By the end of the 10-day camp, however, it is assumed that all traces of medication were removed from the body, giving true readings. The results for the diabetes and asthma students who completed medical testing are tabulated in this table.

Patient	31.1.1983	8.2.1983
1	F 75	F 70
	PP102	PP 90
	U nil	U nil
2	F 120	F 102
	PP162	PP132
	U nil	U nil
3	F 140	F 110
	PP195	PP142
	U 3+	U nil
4	F 182	F 152
	PP195	PP174
	U 3+	U +
5	F 304	F 305
	PP450	PP387
	U 3+	U 3+
6	F 168	F 146
	PP210	PP168
	U 3+	U nil

F = fasting
PP = postprandial
U = urine sugar; blood sugar in mg%

Discussion on diabetes

All patients experienced some form of improvement. It should be noted that patient 5 was an insulin dependent

250

diabetic, unwilling to take insulin and also not well controlled by insulin. In this type of situation long-term yogic management and follow-up is necessary. However, in this trial, as in the previous trial from Kanpur, this did not prove possible despite the excellent hospital facilities available. The problem here appears to be motivational and linked somehow to the Indian social situation.

Asthma

Fifteen asthmatics were measured with lung function tests at the M.G.M. Medical College before and after the course. They ranged from mild, seasonal to severe asthma. The results are given below.

	PFR		FEV	
Patient	Before	After	Before	After
1	200	240	59	59
2	200	220	58	62
3	275	420	84	76
4	340	360	64	64
5	450	510	200	100
6	450	500	81	81
7	300	320	53	53
8	220	220	69	68
9	200	270	92	92
10	550	580	86	90
11	150	220	53	54
12	340	550	75	73
13	410	460	63	72
14	550	550	72	65
15	150	250	67	67

PFR = pulmonary flow rate litres/minute
FEV = forced expiration volume as percentage

Discussion

Dr Venkatesh, one of the doctors helping to organize the medical side of the camp, stated, "At the beginning of the course it was observed that the hall was echoing with the coughing, wheezing and sneezing of the participants. What was amazing was that by about the fourth or fifth day the hall gave an atmosphere of silence and serenity, no more coughing, sneezing or wheezing.

"Lung function tests were performed at the M.G.M. Medical College. Tests were done before and after the course and improvement in almost all the cases was noticed. It was seen that the younger the subject the better the result.

"Fasting and postprandial readings of the blood sugar were taken before and after the course. A marked fall in blood sugar was seen in the majority of cases.

"Recordings of blood pressure were taken before and after the course. Here again, an appreciable fall was noted. In a few cases there was no difference.

"Seeing these results one is naturally led to the conclusion that these practices really help."

ASTHMA, DIABETES AND HYPERTENSION CAMP, BEGUSARAI

An asthma, diabetes and hypertension camp was held at the Yoga Sansthan, Begusarai (Bihar), from 1st to 21st June 1984. The Indian Medical Association, Begusarai Branch, lent close co-operation in assessing the medical condition and effects of yoga for each aspirant.

This camp spurred great interest in yoga in the community, and the doctors present during the camp felt that the results were so impressive that they warranted a much deeper, controlled study of yoga. We feel that the results of this camp were particularly good because it was held within an ashram environment.

Diabetes research

The results of four patients of the diabetes group are given below. There is obvious improvement in all four cases and a dramatic improvement in patients 1 and 4.

Patient	Before		After	
1	F208	PP247	F 90	PP 94
2	F128	PP213	F-	PP171
3	F112	PP143	F108	PP134
4	F216	PP412	F124	PP241

F = fasting,
PP = postprandial; all results are in mg%

Asthma research

The objective improvement in the asthmatics was gauged by white blood cell count (WCC), the eosinophil level (E) as a percentage of the WCC, and the clinical picture as judged by a qualified medical practitioner.

Most of the asthmatics felt subjective improvement until halfway through the course when the unexpectedly early change from hot season to monsoon caused temperatures to drop precipitously, resulting in most of the 10 asthmatics developing fevers and acute asthma attacks.

It had been our intention to teach the group yoga before the monsoon started, to prepare them for the drop in temperature and the change in season. We have previously seen that, when people learn yoga techniques and develop preliminary skills, they can handle various stresses and strains such as change of season much more easily when they come. Despite these difficulties the objective results in the 4 students who remained in the course despite acute attacks and fever were very encouraging. All

Patient	Before	After
1 WCC	14,600	6,600
E	56	42
2 WCC	10,300	7,800
E	6.4	2
3 WCC	10,000	6,500
E	7	1
4 WCC		
E	23	15

253

4 patients had drops in their WCC and eosinophils, which indicates yoga's capacity to influence the immune system.

General conclusion

All of the camps proved to be successful therapeutically and engendered a great deal of enthusiasm both within the community and medical profession. On the whole the results were very encouraging and many of the people concerned requested repeated camps on a yearly basis.

Several points and difficulties emerged in these trials. The first was that many of the participants expected that they would be cured by the end of the camp and that further practice would not be necessary. This is a common problem in many therapeutic situations and it was necessary to explain to the students that what they were learning was the beginning of their yogic career and that time is required to develop skill in practice, purification, strength and health.

In all these camps it was necessary to explain basic concepts of health and to define health as an on-going process requiring constant maintenance rather than as something that we can achieve and then forget about. The realization that change is natural and that we are constantly growing is important in regaining health because it introduces the idea that we have to change those parts of our lifestyles, habits and attitudes which were causing our disease in the first place. It also means that we have to continue our yoga practices regularly and consistently.

One of the great problems encountered in these trails was that of long-term follow-up. For some reason this seemed to be almost impossible, though we have been in touch with several of the more enthusiastic participants who have reported continuous and progressive improvement with constant yoga practice.

Another important point which emerged was that an ashram environment or some kind of live-in situation is important in order to standardize variables such as diet and lifestyle, and also to allow participants to experience deep relaxation away from the problems, worries and tensions that inevitably build up in the home, work and life in general.

In those camps in which a live-in situation was possible, the overall subjective and objective results were much better. This may indicate that ashram living on its own, with a relaxed yogic lifestyle and a few simple asana and pranayama, may be enough to eliminate certain diseases. Further trials will require controls to account for this factor.

With the experience we have gained from these camps, research continues at the Ganga Darshan research facilities where we can regulate and control laboratory studies, diet and other variables. In this way we hope to obtain clear and scientifically definitive results.

One point definitely emerges from the studies done in the past in our yoga camps for asthma, diabetes and high blood pressure, and that is that yoga definitely has a lot to offer people at the level of physical and mental well-being. Apart from the objective improvements, most of the participants left feeling improved and better able to manage their condition. We are confident that people with these conditions no longer have to think of themselves as being burdened with an incurable, life-threatening disease for the rest of their lives and that more people should seek guidance in yoga, in combination with professional medical guidance, in order to rid themselves of these chronic degenerative and psychosomatic conditions while they are in the early stages.

33

Clinical Trials

The following chapter is a brief summary of the available literature reporting on the yogic treatment of asthma and diabetes from various institutions in India plus one report from Australia and one from Japan. These reports share the common denominator of various combinations and permutations of asana, pranayama, relaxation and hatha yoga shatkarma, as the basis of their treatment program.

Australia

M.K. Tandon reported from the Thoracic Division of the Repatriation General Hospital, Hollywood, Western Australia, on the 11 cases of severe, irreversible, chronic obstructive airways disease patients, ages ranging from 53–65 years and having chronic bronchitis with or without pulmonary emphysema, who were given training in yogic breathing exercises and postures.[1] A control group of 11 patients, ages ranging from 52–64 years, were given physiotherapy breathing exercises. Follow-ups with pulmonary function tests, exercise tolerance and inquiry into symptoms were conducted at monthly intervals for nine months.

The yoga group performed significantly better on objective tests of exercise tolerance though there was no change in lung function tests. Tandon states that yoga training helped to change the breathing pattern of the patients to a slower and deeper pattern, which helped them to tolerate higher work loads. The yoga group recovered more quickly after exertion and could control an attack of severe shortness of breath using breathing exercises without resorting to medical help. They claimed to have a definite improvement in their overall chest condition. These results are remarkable and very significant, especially from the asthmatic point of view because asthma is also a mild, reversible obstructive airways disease. If such good subjective results can be had in elderly people with severe respiratory obstruction, then the application of yoga for asthma is of great benefit.

Bombay

Dr M.V. Divekar, Professor and Head of the Department of Medicine, L.T.M. Medical College and Hospital, Sion, Bombay, reports on a trial of 52 chronic, uncomplicated diabetics with more than 3 years history of the disease.[2] They were all less than 55 years old and all were on drugs and dietary restrictions prior to coming to yoga. These people practised asana for four months and afterwards were assessed for weight loss and blood sugar. The blood sugar level dropped to normal in 18 cases of insulin dependent diabetes, and 20 cases using oral drugs. This necessitated decreased dosages of medication. Two patients totally stopped their drugs.

Divekar also studied obesity in 38 patients and found 2–4 kilogram weight reduction in 18 cases, 4–6 kilogram reduction in two cases and 8 kilogram reduction in one case. All patients in the trial experienced subjective relief from tension headaches and indigestion and experienced feelings of lightness and enhanced well-being.

It is interesting to note that good results were obtained in this study using only asana and a little pranayama. People have reported to us that by asana alone they were unable to eradicate diabetes and eliminate the need for drugs. However, from our experience, as soon as laghoo shankha-prakshalana, pranayama and yoga nidra are incorporated

257

into a yogic sadhana program, vast improvement is experienced at all levels. The study by Divekar points out the effectiveness of asana when practised regularly over a period of time.

Exercise is known to be important in the treatment of diabetes and certain cases respond to this alone. However, yoga asana are not exercises in the traditional sense; they are postures. Divekar states, "It may be criticized that yoga therapy is nothing but physical exercise. This is not so; yoga asana are meant for physical suppleness and mental relaxation. Our patients at the end of 30 minutes yoga therapy did not feel tired or exhausted. On the contrary, they felt relaxed when they did it in the right manner."

Divekar has also conducted trials on asthma. The 170 cases were from 7–72 years of age and did not take medication. The students learned pranayama (sectional breathing, hasta mudra and mukha bhastrika, forcing techniques and healing breath by chest tapping) in six lessons and were tested before and after classes and after 3–6 weeks for lung function (maximum ventilatory volume, forced expiratory volume, vital capacity and peak expiratory flow). Of those who practised regularly, there was excellent improvement in 64 cases (43.3%) and moderate improvement in 59 cases (39.9%). Divekar states, "This striking result of yoga therapy calls for greater application in correction of asthma."

The Yoga Institute of Santa Cruz, Bombay, performed a four-month study of 23 asthma patients and found an 87% rate of moderate improvement or better.[3] In 1976 the Institute made a follow-up of former patients and 38 cases followed up over an average of 7 years indicated positive improvement in 31 patients, 30 of whom were all practising yoga.[4] Most of these people reported changes in daily routine, food habits and attitudes. One of the patients in this study showed some radiographic evidence of greater diaphragmatic excursion.

Jaipur

The Yogic Treatment-cum-Research Centre in Jaipur, Rajasthan, run by Swami Anandananda, reported in their Progress Report from August 1961 to December 1980, good results in the treatment of asthma and diabetes.

A total of 533 cases of diabetes had been treated and of these 407 had completed treatment. Out of these 267 (65.4%) had improved or been cured and 140 (34.4%) had not improved.

Out of a total of 472 asthma patients seen, 348 had completed treatment and of these 219 (62.9%) had improved or been cured, 97 (27.9%) had not improved and 32 (9.2%) were doubtful.

In another paper from Jaipur, Varandani, Anandananda and Dharmveer reported on the treatment of 283 diabetic patients through yoga.[5] Ages ranged from 14–68 years and they had suffered from diabetes for one to more than ten years. Twenty-three percent of patients left without finishing the course.

The subjects were divided into the following groups:
1. Mild (30%), with fasting blood sugar up to 120 milligrams percent.
2. Moderate, up to 180 milligrams percent.
3. Severe, greater than 180 milligrams percent.

It is interesting to note that only 32% of subjects had a positive hereditary history while 58% were judged to have significant emotional or psychic factors contributing to their disease. The typical personality in this group was that of a highly intelligent, sensitive, brooding nature, with some sort of maladjustment to the environment.

Blood sugar was recorded before and after the subjects practised kunjal, vastra dhauti, shankhaprakshalana, asana and nauli. It was found that 25% of the 283 patients responded completely to yoga therapy and blood sugar levels reached normal limits with no sugar in the urine. Of these, 19 received a test carbohydrate diet which they tolerated without rise of blood sugar.

Twenty-seven percent of patients showed great improvement in their blood sugar and though they did not reach normal levels, they gave up all medication and their symptoms were alleviated. A further 25% did not respond to yoga therapy and these were either juvenile or long duration cases who had been using insulin over a long period of time or were an older age group and could not perform the practices properly.

This trial was carried out in an ashram atmosphere and the authors felt that this helped to contribute to the removal of stress and tension from the lives of the students. The factors involved were change of environment, regularity of daily routine, yogic atmosphere and group support, and counselling by the swami and the doctor in charge. The combination of asana and pranayama plus the ashram environment is thought to have led to the healing and rejuvenation of the students.

Japan

Dr John Goyeche, Associate Professor of Psychology at Kurume University Medical School, Kurume, Japan, reports that out of 10 asthma patients treated over a 3 year period with yoga and other therapeutic treatments, 7 showed marked improvement with complete disappearance of symptoms in some cases.[6] The 3 remaining cases also showed some improvement. Follow-up of 3 cases indicates further improvement through yoga. All patients and most of their physicians have testified to the great value of yoga practice in treatment. Goyeche writes that, "The process seen in most of these patients is first one of emotional discharge such as anger and crying, and then development of the ability to lose themselves in concentration, which is followed by the relief of symptoms. Most patients claim that they learn to control attacks by yoga methods, especially the breathing techniques, which reduce anxiety at the time of attack, although this is obviously a gross over-simplification of a profound psychophysiological transformation."

Kanyakumari

R. Nagarathna and H.R. Nagendra of the Vivekananda Kendra Yoga Therapy and Research Centre, Kanyakumari, South India, reported good results in 15 patients with diabetes. [7] The patients had diabetes for from 1–28 years. One insulin dependent diabetic had a non-healing ulcer on her foot which healed with the yogic practices taught: shatkarma, asana and pranayama. After 3 months follow-up, there was significant weight reduction. The authors state that, "These significant improvements... (are) mainly due to reduction of weight and the release of stresses by deep relaxation technique."

Out of 46 patients with asthma there was significant reduction in severity of attacks, duration of attacks, number of attacks per week, nasal allergies and dose of medication. The authors felt that these improvements came from deep relaxation, removal of panic and the development of internal awareness and stamina by yogic practices.

Pune

M.V. Bhole from Kaivalyadhama, Pune, reported a 76% rate of cure or improvement by both clinical and laboratory assessment in 114 asthma cases treated only by yoga over one year.[8] All the people who persisted in their yogic practices showed some improvement and attacks of asthma could usually be prevented by yoga practices alone without resorting to drugs.

R.V. Ranade of the Yoga Vidya Dham, Pune, reported good improvement in 7 out of 22 asthma patients, fair improvement in 12 cases and little improvement in 3 cases. At 6 and 12-month follow-up, there was sustained improvement. They also reported a good improvement in 16 cases of diabetes studied.

Tirupathi

Rajyalakshmi at Tirupathi reported that out of 20 cases of diabetes treated at the Indian Institute of Research in Yoga

261

and Allied Sciences, 15 achieved a good response to yoga, 3 cases had a fair response and in 2 cases only slight response was found.[9]

T.M. Srinivasin and B.L. Meti measured 12 asthmatics doing daily yoga practice from 30–60 days as in-patients in the yogic hospital at Tirupathi.[10] Half the patients showed marked improvement and displayed increases in both vital capacity and forced expiratory volume which was maintained over a three-month follow-up period. Three patients (25%) showed no improvement.

Varanasi

R. Singh, R.M. Shettiwar and K.N.Udupa reported from Benares Hindu University on 85 cases of diabetes treated at their yoga centre.[11] These were all early onset diabetes with no complications. Complete relief was found in 30%, substantial relief in 31.6% partial relief in 28.3% no relief in 11.6% and only 2 of the patients deteriorated.

Asthma was also studied and out of 115 cases, 22.6% had complete relief, 28.3% substantial relief, 35.7% partial relief, 13.9% no relief and only one person in the group had deteriorated.

The authors stated, "All these patients had prolonged medical treatment which proved unsatisfactory. After practice of yoga, in many patients the drug requirement was considerably reduced and some of them could do well without anything."

Others

N.S. Vahia, a psychiatrist, has claimed a 93% improvement in 15 patients being treated by yoga therapy over 6 weeks in a hospital out-patient study.[12] Clinical improvement was significantly associated with increased concentration capacity and it was felt that meditation practice improved the effect of asana and pranayama. The therapy, which was aimed at increasing internal experience and self-awareness, reduced anxiety scores more than drug therapy.

262

A.K. Choudhary and his colleagues at the Indian Institute of Yoga at Patna, Bihar, reported that of 11 patients with diabetes 9 patients were cured and 2 juvenile diabetics improved. The 7 asthma patients studied were all said to be completely cured.

Rugmini and Sinha have also reported the beneficial effects of yoga therapy on diabetes.[13]

Conclusion

All the trials above give a clear indication that yoga therapy is of real benefit in treating asthma and diabetes. Only one study showed that out of 200 cases, 3 cases reported deleterious effects[11], and to our knowledge this is a very rare finding in yoga therapy, especially when the practices are being taught under expert guidance. It usually occurs because the individuals concerned do not follow instructions properly. On the contrary, most authors agreed that, even when the yoga practices did not relieve the asthma or diabetes completely, the patients reported subjective improvement and enhanced well-being.

The reports given in this chapter are remarkable in that most of the patients involved in the trials showed improvement without requiring medication or other forms of therapy. These were patients who, for the most part, had been unsuccessfully treated by orthodox medical means. These trials justify further work into yoga therapy and justify referral by doctors of their patients to a good yoga teacher in order to incorporate yoga into the orthodox medical regimes.

We hope that more such trials will be performed to settle the question of yoga's role in chronic psychosomatic and degenerative disease as soon as possible and we intend to do our part in this. This is important, not just to give yoga scientific respectability, but also to give more doctors and healing professionals better tools in the battle against disease and, more importantly, to give the patients a better chance of good health and a normal, happy and full life.

34

How Yoga Works

The discovery that yoga is of value in treating diseases such as high blood pressure, diabetes and asthma has inspired doctors and researchers engaged in the battle against such diseases to perform properly controlled trials in order to explain yoga's capacity to effect body and mind in clear, logical and scientific terms. Yoga's ability to affect the mind and body has been researched from two main points of view: firstly, the capacity of yoga to deal with and affect individuals, and secondly, its capacity to deal with a disease situation. In this chapter we will deal with yoga's influence on normal people and present certain studies which show how yoga can lower blood sugar and affect our metabolism in the normal situation. The results of these trials can be used to understand yoga better in the disease situation.

Research at Varanasi

Drs Udupa, Singh and Settiwar studied 12 normal, healthy males aged between 20 and 26 years.[1] They learned asana, pranayama and hatha yoga shatkarma, one hour daily for 6 months. Physiological measurements were made at the beginning and at the end of 3 months and 6 months. The general, overall findings were:

• There was decreased body weight and abdominal girth. This is very important from the point of view of health in general and diabetes in particular.

- There was decreased respiratory rate combined with increased vital capacity of the lungs, breath holding time and chest expansion, indicating overall improvement in lung function and is important from the point of view of general vitality and in the asthmatic situation.
- An insignificant tendency to lower pulse rate and blood pressure was noted. Also under physical stress there was a reduced tendency to increase the pulse rate. The rate of fall in vital capacity and the rate of increase in mental fatigue also decreased indicating an overall increase in stamina and resistance to stress.
- Increased secretion of the adrenal hormones as evidenced by the increased secretion of 17-hydroxycorti- costeroids, 17-ketosteroids and vanillyl mandelic acid (VMA) was found. From this we would expect an increased blood sugar in response to increased adrenal activity; however, the opposite was true.
- Blood sugar levels fell significantly.
- Blood cholesterol levels also fell significantly.
- Serum protein levels increased significantly.

Udupa and his colleagues have confirmed these findings in repeated trials in which the following were also noted:
- Dominant alpha brain wave activity indicating relaxation.
- Improved performance in memory quotient and neuroticism levels.
- Decreased mental fatigue.
- Increased protein-bound iodine indicating an effect on the thyroid gland.
- Increased testosterone in urine indicating an effect on the gonads.
- Decreased erythrocyte acetylcholine and cholinesterase levels.[2-4]

Udupa studied the breathing techniques of ujjayi (performed for 7 minutes) followed by bhastrika (for 10 minutes), a highly energizing and stimulating sequence of pranayama, and again showed increased adrenal gland secretion and decreased blood sugar.[5]

In studies of vipassana meditation the opposite results to those found in asana and pranayama were found in some secretions[6], e.g. there was a drop in plasma cortisol and urinary corticosteroids as well as urinary nitrogen, and an increase in erythrocyte acetylcholine and cholinesterase levels, as well as plasma histaminase and catecholamines.

Jevning and his colleagues have also shown that during certain forms of relaxative meditation there is a decrease in plasma cortisol, consistent with the complete inhibition of adrenocortical activity in long-term practitioners during meditation.[7] This was found to be unrelated to sleep during meditation practice. This is probably due to the complete inhibition of the pituitary-adrenal activity.

Michaels and her colleagues reported that relaxative medi-tation and simple eyes closed relaxation both reduced cortisol levels.[8] The control group showed a significant rise in cortisol following the venipuncture whereas meditators did not, indicating that meditation neutralizes the stress response.

These findings have very important ramifications from the psychosomatic point of view. They show us that it is possible to influence the pituitary gland, the adrenals, thyroid and gonads, either directly or indirectly through yoga. They indicate that through yoga it is possible to influence, mani-pulate and modulate the total endocrine system, metabolism, and ultimately the total personality and level of well-being.

Udupa states, "This enhanced adrenocortical activity makes these subjects competent to resist stress and probably in such subjects stress may not produce instantaneous endo-crine and metabolic changes which may usually be associated with certain undesirable effects. The physiological studies done on these subjects have also shown significant evidence of development of resistance against physical stress. In spite of increased adrenocortical activity, no increased breakdown of proteins has been noted, which indicates compatibility of the enhanced adrenocortical activity in these subjects."

The results of this trial are interesting because with an increased level of adrenal hormones one would expect to see an increased blood sugar and decreased protein level. However, the opposite was observed and these findings have been confirmed by the reports of H.S. Nayar which will be described in the next section.

Udupa and his colleagues feel that yoga postures may vitalize the body's internal activity leading to various changes, such as the drop in blood sugar. They feel that the drop in blood glucose and the increased serum protein levels, despite increased activity of the adrenal cortex, support the possibility of an active insulin-like mechanism counteracting the catabolic effects of the corticosteroids. No insulin measurements were made in this trial, however, more trials will be needed to sort out this complex and important point.

Research at Delhi

H.S. Nayar and his colleagues have confirmed the findings of Udupa.[9] A 6-month controlled study of 30 healthy was conducted, which included asana, pranayama and meditation (with emphasis on asana), with the following results:
1. Decreased heart rate and blood pressure and decreased lung ventilation and oxygen consumption which indicate a more relaxed, hypometabolic condition.
2. Increased alpha brain waves which indicate a relaxed state.
3. Increased net mechanical efficiency and decreased oxygen consumption during submaximal exercise plus no change in blood lactic acid levels, which indicate a greater degree of physical fitness.
4. Blood glucose, cholesterol and lipoprotein ratio decreased and the authors feel that this is due to increased parasympathetic activity.
5. Increased levels of the enzymes monoamine oxydase and plasma cholinasterase with decreased dopamine B-hydroxylase indicating a more relaxed, parasympathetic dominant state.
6. Increased adrenal gland secretion was evidenced by increased 17-hydroxycorticosteroids and 17-ketosteroids in the urine.

7. Increased levels of haemoglobin, hematocrit, platelet count, fibrinolytic activity, platelet aggregation time and activated partial thromboplastin plus decreased plasma fibrinogen levels indicating a decreased tendency for blood clotting and less chance for intravascular thrombosis and artherosclerosis.

8. When exposed to cold, the yoga subject showed less vasoconstriction than controls, indicating less sympathetic activity and improved thermo-regulating efficiency. This is possibly due to improved functioning of the hypothalamic regulatory mechanisms in the brain.

The authors state, "Regular yogic practice for 6 months has been observed to improve physiological and biochemical functions of the body... (and) indicate a trend of gradual shift of autonomic equilibrium toward relative parasympathodominance by reduction of sympathetic activity... The practice of hatha yoga, pranayama and different bandha have specific influence on autonomic functions, activity of CNS and endocrine system... The stable autonomic equilibrium and relative hypometabolic states achieved by yogic practice may be the scientific basis for the claim that yogic practice endows perfect physical and mental health."

Research at Pondicherry

K. S. Gopal and his colleagues have studied 22 students practising asana, pranayama, mudra, bandha and kriya, and have found that after 6 months training there was:

1. Decreased blood sugar in 11 students.
2. Decreased blood cholesterol in 12 students.
3. Increased total protein in 7 students, increased albumin in 10 students and decreased globulin in 6 students.[10]

The authors state that, "In our view, the decreased blood sugar could have been brought about by increased peripheral utilization of glucose... Whatever changes have occurred at the end of six months, they are desirable ones... These beneficial, biochemical effects suggest the possible application of hatha yogic practices for the prevention of diseases like diabetes mellitus, arthosclerosis, obesity and the like."

Summary
These trials on asana, pranayama, hatha yoga, relaxation and meditation throw light on the mechanism of action of yoga techniques. One thing emerges clearly, that yoga leads us to a more relaxed state of enhanced physical health, stamina and endurance, and overall physical and mental well being. It is still too early to make any definitive statement on yoga's capacity to affect the body; many more trials will be required to sort out the many variables involved and to develop standardization. In the trials reported here, various different techniques have been used and even when the same techniques were used, we cannot say that they were performed in the same way and with the same degree of proficiency.

Another point to consider is that certain techniques are said to bring about a generalized balancing of body processes, for example, sarvangasana (the shoulder stand) is said to be able both to reduce hyperthyroidism and activate a sluggish hypothyroid situation. Nadi shodhana pranayama is another neutral type of exercise which aims at rebalance. Bhastrika pranayama or a vigorous asana routine tends to raise the metabolism, blood pressure, and so on, and there are other practices specifically to lower it.

We should also note that we cannot consider any one result on its own but must rather view them within the total psychophysiological context of the individual, and must evaluate both the objective and subjective points of view. There are many variables which must be considered, for example, if the asana is static or dynamic; whether breathing, mudra or bandha are used; duration of and skill in practice, and many more.

Basically the practices of asana and pranayama had the following effects which together signify, increased physical health and mental relaxation.

- Decreased body weight.
- Decreased breathing rate and increased breathing efficiency.
- Decreased heart rate and blood pressure.
- Decreased blood sugar and cholesterol levels and increased serum protein level.
- Decreased tendency to blood clotting.
- Better exercise tolerance.
- Decreased reaction to cold exposure.
- Increased adrenal, gonadal and thyroid gland secretion.
- Increased alpha brain waves (relaxation).
- Improved memory.
- Decreased mental fatigue and neuroticism.

Certain meditation and relaxation techniques indicated decreased secretion from the adrenal cortex and past trials indicated that a generalized hypometabolic situation occurs.

In terms of understanding how these techniques could work in the diabetic situation, they would help in the following way:
1. Increased weight loss.
2. Lowered blood sugar, either by insulin activation and/or decreased sympathetic activity and/or better tissue utilization (probably a combination of all three).
3. Decreased mental tension.

All three are important factors in dealing with the diabetic, high blood sugar situation.

In the asthma situation yoga would help by:
1. Improving lung function directly, making the lungs stronger and more efficient.
2. Relaxation of the mental tension which often leads to an attack.
3. Raising blood cortisone levels (instead of using external sources of cortisone, the yogic practices would stimulate the body's own internal secretions).

More research is required to verify these theories; however, it is important to realize the directions such research should take.

Stimulating the chakras

The research to date suggests that a balanced program of asana, pranayama and relaxation/meditation would stimulate and balance the nervous, endocrine and metabolic activity. Perhaps this is what the yogis meant when they said that even asanas stimulate the chakras, e.g. increased adrenal gland activity indicates enhanced manipura chakra activity. Although there was increased adrenal gland secretion, there was no rise in blood sugar or signs of mental or physical stress, as would be expected. Rather there were concomitant signs of mental relaxation and physical health. This indicates that the overall readiness of the body to handle stress is improved and that due to regular asana practice the basal resistance of the body is better. A yogi would state that when manipura is turned on, the body becomes healthy and glows with prana and is better able to resist disease.

These studies show us that we can affect not only manipura but also swadhisthana, vishuddhi and ajna chakras.

The importance of auto-regulation

Perhaps the most important point to realize here is that yoga makes it possible to manipulate the internal physical and mental environment without the aid of drugs. Specific techniques are claimed to have specific effects, and this is the basis of a scientific system.

Yoga, therefore emerges as a method by which we can stimulate and regulate the internal body processes, without the need for drugs and other external agents. This confers a great sense of independence, autonomy and self-confidence on the yogi. As we become more adept at yoga, we can begin to sense which practices we need to do in order to bring about balance in our own body. For example, a little more asana and pranayama to speed things up, or a little more relaxation and meditation to slow things down. By adjusting the various ratios, rhythms, duration and timing of our practice, we are able to self-regulate our internal mechanisms and thereby gain perfect physical and mental health.

271

35

Research on Bronchial Asthma at Raipur Medical College

G.B. Gupta (lecturer), G.C. Sepaha (professor and head of department), I. Menone (postgraduate student), S.K. Tiwari (reader) Department of Medicine, J.N.M. Medical College, Raipur, M.P., India.

Yogic practices are very ancient and provide the practitioner with control over certain functions of the body including the autonomic nervous system. It is claimed that one can also control certain metabolic/endocrine processes so as to enter the state of superconsciousness. Though yoga is basically not a method of treating disease, one can find citations in literature advocating its curative and prophylactic values in certain diseases like hypertension, diabetes mellitus, bronchial asthma, peptic ulcer, etc.

Normally sensory perception of external episodes leads to emotional and mental responses. As a result there are hypothalmic/pituitary/autonomic/adrenal axis responses which often are reflected in physiological changes manifested by sweating, tachycardia, palpitation, raised blood pressure, etc. and in some patients broncho-constriction (possibly only in asthmatics).

Yogic techniques can be used to bring about a state of relaxation. Relaxation means non-perception and/or non-responsiveness to external sensory inputs. By yogic techniques, if they bring about relaxation, the above-mentioned physiochemical changes may be intercepted. Thus yoga helps in modifying the emotional and mental

272

responses, mediated by the hypothalmic axis, which may normalize disturbed homeostasis.

In 1978, a study was planned to observe the effects of some yogic practices (advocated for bronchial asthma) on ventilatory function tests and clinical features in cases of bronchial asthma.

Material and methods

Twenty-seven cases of both sexes, 19 extrinsic and 8 intrinsic were divided into 3 groups:

- *Group 1*: 12 patients taking drugs only at the time of an attack.
- *Group 2*: 11 patients controlled with bronchodilators and having recurrence on omission of drugs.
- *Group 3*: 4 patients whose attacks were not controlled with adequate doses of bronchodilators.

All cases were trained in yogic practices by specialist yoga teachers at Raipur Yogavidyalaya for a period of 6 weeks after which they continued these practices in their homes. Yogic practices included jala neti, kunjal kriya, vastra dhauti and pranayama. During yogic practices patients were not taking any medicines. Bronchodilators were given only at the time of an acute attack.

Forced vital capacity (FVC), forced expiratory volume in one second (FEV), FEV/FVC ratio, and maximum breathing capacity (MBC) were studied prior to, at weekly intervals during yogic practices and at the termination of the study on the sixth week. A spirograph curve was used to estimate these ventilatory function tests. Clinical assessment of improvement was done by arbitrary grading of relief in symptoms and signs before and after yogic practices.

Observation and discussion

Three cases discontinued the practices within one week, hence are excluded from further report. 90% (9 cases) of group 1 and 60% (6 cases) of group 2 did not get any attack of asthma during the program. They showed some symptomatic and ventilatory function improvement. These 15 patients showing improvement had a history of recurrent coryza with asthma. They had subsequent reduction in the frequency and duration of asthmatic attacks. Doses of drugs required to control these attacks were reduced by 30–40% at the end of the 6 weeks course of yogic practices. Patients described certain additional advantages like gain in stamina, greater capacity to concentrate, more desire to work and feeling at ease.

Similar benefits like subjective feelings of well-being, confidence and ability to accomplish modest but previously impossible tasks were reported in exercise programs by Nicholos and his associates (1970). Significant physical and emotional benefits were also reported in a swimming program for asthmatics by Fitch and his colleagues (1976).

Twenty-nine percent (7 out of 24) cases had persistence of bronchospasm during the practice period for which bronchodilators had to be given. Two cases in group 3 did not show any improvement and they went into status asthmaticus requiring hospital management.

Seventeen patients had extrinsic and seven patients had intrinsic type of asthma. No difference was detected in the degree of improvement in these two types of asthmatics.

Patients of group 1 showed 34.23% and 15% improvement in FEV and FVC values respectively at the end of the trial period. FEV/FVC ratio changed from 64.33 to 67.33. Group 2 patients had 20% improvement in FVC and 9% improvement in FEV at the end of six weeks. Group 3 patients showed no significant improvement in VFT (ventilatory function test) during or at the end of the trial period. Nicholos and his associates (1970) also reported insignificant changes in pulmonary function tests of similar (group 3) cases after the exercise program.

Cases belonging to group 1 included early cases with mild asthma and group 2 included later cases with moderate severity of asthma. These had some symptomatic and ventilatory function improvement with yogic practices. This

274

suggests that yogic practices are generally beneficial only in the early cases with mild or moderate severity of the disease rather than in severe, persistent forms of asthma. To obtain maximum benefits from these practices, it is therefore advisable to start them at the earliest stage.

The precise way in which these yogic practices exert their effects are not known. Some of them possibly act by altering the reflex response of the vagus nerve. Amongst the four practices, kunjal kriya and vastra dhauti seem to have greater reflex effect on the respiratory system. Pranayama involves breath retention during which alteration in $pCo2$ and pH occurs. This might be acting in one way or another. These yogic practices possibly exert some effects (which are not understood) on the hypothalamus.

Yogic techniques do not involve muscular exercises, neither do they cause increase in oxygen consumption. On the other hand, it is found that there is a fall in temperature. This may be enhanced by perspiration which commonly accompanies kunjal kriya. It is well known that reduced muscular activity, hypothermia, and decreased oxygen consumption lead to reduction in metabolic processes. Whether this could contribute towards some beneficial effects in asthma can only be decided by experimental designs. From the four yogic practices, which one proves to be superior, can only be said when studies on individual practices are conducted. Work on this is under progress in our department.

Two features observed in these patients deserve mention. Firstly, those who performed yogic practices in groups were more benefited than those who did it alone. It seems that being in a group helps the patient to forget all his problems which are important psychological precipitating factors. A person gets some sort of psychological satisfaction when he knows that he is not the only one suffering, or there may be a sense of well-being derived from mutual sympathy. Secondly, those who accepted yoga keenly and easily were benefited more than those who resisted and did not show

275

much interest in it. Motivation, especially when senior physicians prescribe and encourage, has an indirect, reassuring effect. Additional benefits dependent on placebo effects, easy acceptability, group therapy and religious beliefs, etc., of a psychological nature must also be taken into account.

Asthma is an episodic syndrome. To draw firm conclusions from a short-range study of 6 to 12 weeks only, is not possible, especially considering the chances of spontaneous and natural remissions in early and moderate cases. Though spectacular improvement did not occur in any case, it is obvious that the yogic practices are useful in the early cases with mild to moderate severity of the disease. Persons chosen for yogic practices should have a high degree of motivation, easy acceptability and no other associated illness. As far as possible, yogic practices should be done in a group, preferably by forming small clubs for asthmatics.

Benefits in the respiratory functions, additional symptomatic advantages like sense of well being, comradeship of group energy, and training for better exercise tolerance gives support to the idea that if these practices are done early and persistently, benefits may accrue. Whether a chronic disabling state can thereby be prevented cannot be said at present, but it is a distinct possibility.

Summary

Ventilatory function test (VFT) in 27 cases of bronchial asthma was studied before, during and at the end of a six-week course of yogic practices. Three patients left the study. 62.5% of the patients showed some improvement in VFT and clinical features. These were cases of early disease with mild to moderate severity. Patients with severe and persistent asthma showed no improvement. No difference in the improvement was observed between extrinsic and the intrinsic types.

36

Diabetes Camp
at Calcutta Ashram

Dr N.C. Panda, Burla Medical College (Orissa)

In 1976 the International Diabetes Federation meeting was held in India for the first time. During the meeting, however, it became evident that adequate systematic research had not yet been carried out in the area of diabetes and yoga. I felt that this was unfortunate, as the science of yoga has much to contribute to our medical knowledge. Therefore, I decided to launch a scientific program for diabetics in which the yogic system could be thoroughly tested.

In April 1978 we started the first course at the Bihar School of Yoga Calcutta unit with fifteen diabetics. They were divided into two groups, one which remained on drugs and one which went off drugs. Many of the subjects practised asana but a control group did not. The course was held for one month and results were taken at four intervals. The following are some of the results.

Subject 1 was tested on arrival when his blood sugar level in milligrams per 100 millilitres of blood was 185 fasting/211 after lunch. After one month of asana and diet control his blood sugar was 140 fasting/151 after lunch. Then he was put on asana, diet control and tablets, and the following blood sugar levels were recorded – on two Dalmol tablets twice daily 111 fasting/185 after lunch; on one Dalmol tablet twice daily 104 fasting/106 after lunch. The combination of yoga and medicine proved to be very effective in managing the high blood glucose.

277

Subject 2 was given yoga and diet only. On admission into the ashram his blood sugar was 211/251. By the 25th day it measured 120/135, a normal level.

Subject 3 could not walk or climb stairs on admission. He improved remarkably and after one month was able to climb up and down stairs freely without becoming tired.

Diabetes is mostly due to faulty regulation or insufficiency of insulin. When the insulin levels fall, diabetes occurs. In some cases there may be plenty of insulin but the cells are not able to absorb it. There are many reasons why diabetes occurs so frequently in modern civilization, but it is mostly due to lack of exercise and faulty diet usually combined with overeating. There is also hereditary factor involved, but through the powerful combination of yoga plus a balanced lifestyle, this can be controlled and manifestation of the disease avoided.

Primitive man had a different lifestyle than we have today; he either feasted or fasted. He would hunt until he got something to eat, feast until it was finished, and then fast until he got something else. Today, however, most people do very little physical work, yet they eat all day, every day. Technological development has temporarily solved the food problem and today man is able to have most of the things he wants at any time of the day or night. Modern conveniences have provided us with all the comforts, but at the same time deprived us of exercise and physical work, so necessary for the maintenance of a healthy mind and body. The need for manual labour has greatly decreased while the consumption of rich food has increased.

To make this point more clear, I will tell you about some recent investigations carried out on sand mice. Living in the desert, their natural habitat, they had to work very hard to get their food. When these mice were kept in a cage and fed regularly, they became diabetic within six months. After they were put back in their normal environment the diabetes disappeared. This seems to show that if diet and exercise are balanced, diabetes need not manifest.

278

If any person with diabetes comes to us now, we will tend not to go in for drugs straight away as was the usual protocol five years ago. Instead we will first put him on a proper diet and yogic exercises. At present we have not proved which component of yoga works best, whether it is asana, pranayama or meditation, but we aim to experiment further and come up with more definite answers. I am going to investigate shankhaprakshalana and its effects on both healthy and unhealthy subjects at the Sambalpur ashram, as I feel this is one of the most important components in yoga therapy.

Through our experiments in the field of yoga and diabetes, we have concluded that people with diabetes no longer need to consider themselves as abnormal or permanently incapacitated. Yoga provides a definite means for the diabetic to lead a normal life.

37

Testament to Yoga

Dr Abraham Punnaparambil Kottoyam, Kerala

Personal experience

In 1977, before I sat for my M.D. final examination, I had to undergo a tonsillectomy operation. After the operation I was still disturbed by many mental and physical problems. I had aches and pains all over my body even after the operation. If I sat down to read for any extended time, I had pains in the cervical spine and lower lumbar regions as well as pains all over the body. I was also unable to concentrate. Even three months after the operation my throat always felt uncomfortable. Every morning I would get up with a minimum of twenty or thirty sneezings and running of the nose. So I was taking antihistamines, antibiotics and analgesics, depending upon the symptoms I had. But none of these things completely relieved my complaint.

Later that year, after finishing my degree in general medicine, I went for a short course at Vallabhai Chest Institute in the Department of Allergy and Applied Immunology. I mainly concentrated my study in the field of bronchial asthma. From that time onwards I became aware that allopathic medicine is not able to cure bronchial asthma. It can only alleviate the symptoms.

It was at this point that I received a Bihar School of Yoga magazine from which I learned about jala neti. I started experimenting with this simple nasal cleansing technique, and within one week the effects within my own body were apparent. From that time onwards, I have barely missed a day of this practice.

Secondly, I was cured of trachoma, which is a chronic eye ailment affecting the conjunctiva and giving an almost permanent irritation to the eyes and heaviness of the lids. For the previous ten years I had been applying ointments continuously for this complaint. From the time I started doing neti, I have not applied ointment or drops, but my eyes have been much cooler and have lost all the heaviness. In fact, I have consulted my opthalmology professor and he also told me that all the signs of trachoma have completely disappeared.

Experimental evidence

After these encouraging results upon myself, I decided to try neti with some of my patients. I concentrated mainly on cases of bronchial asthma, and during the last eight or nine months I have seen about 116 cases of both sexes, varying in age from 7–60. I can say with certainty that 80–90% of these people have shown more than 80% improvement during this time.

The severity of asthma ranges from exercise asthma and progresses to the final stage which is called status asthmaticus. Exercise asthma, the least severe form, means that the oxygen supply to the lungs during exercise is inadequate due to the tubes being in a contracted state. During rest these people are all right. Status asthmaticus is the last and most severe stage of asthma in which oxygen demand is not met by the lungs even while resting.

So each patient has to think of his own position along this range and realize that the idea of yogic treatment is to progress gradually to the milder stage of exercise asthma and then on further to the stage of normality.

Using chest measurements at both full inspiration and expiration and recording the difference, we measured the expansion of the lungs. It was found that those asthmatics, around 30–40 years of age, who had a chest expansion of

281

1.5–2 cms. increased this expansion to 4 or 5 cms. after regular performance of yoga practices, including pranayama. In this condition they were completely normal again.

Using a peak Expiratory Flow Meter, I have found that by putting my patients on jala neti and pranayama 70–80% patients have shown 60–70% improvement in lung capacity. Those who improved less were more than 70 years old. The younger patients responded well and have shown almost normal lung measurements.

My research has been very successful and from my experiments I can boldly say that yoga is the best way to eliminate asthma. Modern medicine only relieves the spasm of the bronchioles or removes the congestion of the bronchial tubes, whereas yogic methods bring the individual back to the original state of health.

Appendices

A. Internal Organs

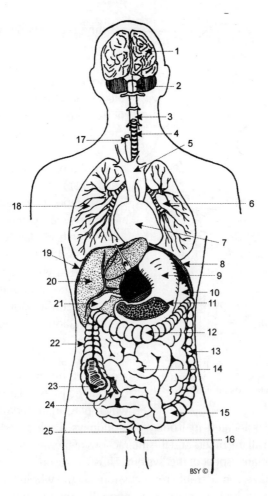

1. Brain	10. Spleen	18. Right Lung
2. Spinal cord	11. Pancreas	19. Diaphragm
3. Vertebral column	12. Transverse colon	20. Liver
4. Trachea	(large intestine)	21. Gall Bladder
5. Aorta	13. Descending colon	22. Ascending colon
6. Left Lung	14. Small intestine	23. Cecum
7. Heart	15. Sigmoid colon	24. Appendix
8. Diaphragm	16. Anus	25. Rectum
9. Stomach	17. Oesophagus	

B. Location of the Endocrine Glands

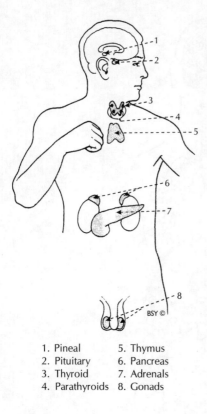

1. Pineal   5. Thymus
2. Pituitary   6. Pancreas
3. Thyroid   7. Adrenals
4. Parathyroids   8. Gonads

Assisting the nervous system is the endocrinal system which consists of chemicals called hormones, secreted by special ductless (endocrine) glands directly into the bloodstream. These hormones are distributed to all parts of the body and govern not only every aspect of metabolism, but also energy levels, temperament, attitude to life and mental power.

The ductless glands are the pituitary and the pineal in the head, the thyroid and parathyroids in the throat, the adrenal glands over the kidneys, and the sex glands (gonads). The pancreas is not properly an endocrine gland, but contains groups of hormone secreting cells called islets of Langerhans, which play an important part in diabetes. It is located in front of the kidneys. Each gland has an influence on all the others and the interactions of the various hormones are an important aspect of this system. Thus any disorder in even one gland will have considerable repercussions on the whole body.

For good health it is necessary to normalize the functioning of the relevant gland and to establish balance and harmony in the system as a whole. The means to do this is the subject matter of this book.

286

C. Location of the Chakras

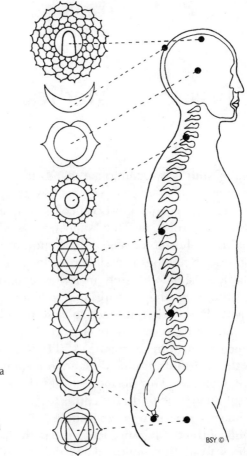

Sahasrara

Bindu

Ajna

Vishuddhi

Anahata

Manipura

Swadhisthana

Mooladhara

BSY ©

Glossary of Medical Terms

Adrenal glands – two endocrine glands located on the top of the kidneys, divided into two sections: cortex and medulla. The former secretes glucocorticoid, mineralocorticoid and some sex steroids, and the latter secretes adrenalin.

Adrenaline – hormone secreted by the adrenal medulla in response to nervous stimulation or lowered blood sugar. It contracts the blood vessels, increases blood pressure, stimulates the heart and prepares the body for intense muscular activity. In addition, it tends to raise the blood sugar level by stimulating release from the liver.

Adrenocorticotrophic hormone (ACTH) – a hormone secreted by the anterior pituitary gland on command from the hypothalamus. This hormone raises the blood sugar level by stimulating the adrenal cortex.

Alimentary – pertaining to digestion.

Alimentary tract – digestive tract; the path that ingested food follows from the mouth, down the oesophagus, into the stomach and intestines, and out of the anus.

Allergy – an unusual bodily chemical response to an ordinary stimulus that is otherwise harmless in similar amounts for most people.

Allergen – any substance which provokes an allergic reaction.

Anaemia – an unhealthy blood condition due to insufficient oxygen-carrying red blood cells, or the cells contain insufficient oxygen-carrying substance (haemoglobin).

Carbon dioxide – a product of respiration which body cells release into the bloodstream after burning oxygen. It is then carried to the lungs and kidneys for excretion.

Cells – the living, active basis of all plant and animal organization, composed of protoplasm contained in a delicate membrane and containing a nucleus.

Cholesterol – an organic chemical which our bodies produce and which we ingest in fatty foods. It is found in bile, the brain, the blood and animal tissues generally.

Chronic – of long and regular duration.

Debility – physical weakness.

Diabetes mellitus – a metabolic disease where the subject is unable to use ingested sugars due to a relative shortage of insulin.

Diaphragm – a large, dome-shaped sheet of muscle between the chest and abdomen.

Dyspnoea – subjective difficulty or distress in breathing, usually associated with disease of the heart or lungs.

Endocrine glands – a group of organs which secrete hormones directly into the blood. These glands are the chief regulators of the body's internal chemical environment.

Excretion – process of elimination of waste matter from the body.

Fat – an organic substance containing glycerol and fatty acids. Usually used to signify food products of animal origin or containing vegetable oils, or a type of soft tissue present in humans and animals. The human body is capable of transforming fat into carbohydrate and carbohydrate into fat (see gluconeogenesis).

Fester – to become infected or gangrenous.

Fibrillation – irregular muscular twitching; can occur in heart.

Fructose – a fruit sugar present in almost all naturally sweet foods.

Galactose – a natural sugar obtained mainly from milk. It is used by the body during childhood for the production of many types of nerve cells.

Gastric – pertaining to the stomach.

Glucocorticoid hormones – a group of hormones secreted by the adrenal cortex which raise the blood sugar level.

Glucose – the major form of carbohydrate, which is stored in the liver and tissues as glycogen.

Gluconeogenesis – chemical synthesis of glucose from proteins and fats in the body.

Glycogenesis – the process of the formation of glycogen from glucose and other sugars in the body.

Glycogenolysis – the breaking down of glycogen into glucose and other substances (e.g. lactic acid).

Hormones – group of chemical substances produced by the glands which regulate the operation of many bodily organs and control the body's metabolism.

Hypertrophy – overgrowth, general increase in organ bulk.

Hypothalamus – a very important section of the midbrain which exercises control over the major internal organs of the body. It is considered to be part of the major functional link between mind and body.

Intercostal muscles – muscles between the ribs.

Insulin – a hormone secreted by the beta cells in the islets of Langerhans in the pancreas. It regulates the carbohydrate metabolism by keeping the blood sugar at a low level, and in its absence the body cannot use ingested sugar.

Islets of Langerhans – a type of cell grouping found in the tail of the pancreas, which produces insulin and secretes it into the blood.

Kidneys – two organs located behind the stomach that secrete urine by removing wastes from the blood.

Liver – large organ situated on the upper right side of the abdomen. It produces bile and converts glucose and lactic acid into glucogen which it stores in large quantities and reconverts to glucose as needed.

Lungs – the major breathing organs located in the chest, containing numerous air cells.

Lymph – colourless alkaline fluid that collects the waste matter not picked up by the bloodstream.

Lymphatic – vessel carrying lymph.

Medulla – the central part of an object or organ.

Medulla oblongata – the prolongation of the spinal cord into the brain. It is about an inch long, cylindrical and enlarged at the upper end.

Metabolism – the combined processes of building up and breaking down substances in the body.

Mucus – slimy substance secreted by certain bodily membranes to keep them moist and to protect internal organs from infection.

Nervous system – control system of the human being; includes the brain, spinal cord, visceral nerves and the superficial nerves. It is the physical mind and the controller of all life processes.

Olfactory bulb – a midbrain formation which is located above the sinuses between the eyebrows. It is the seat of the sense of smell and plays a role in the regulation of the emotions and the stabilization of the functions of the bodily organs.

Overacidity – digestive malfunction characterized by excessive secretions of acid by the digestive glands in the stomach and intestines.

Oxidation – a process of transforming one substance into another in which oxygen is used and energy is liberated. It is one of the prime chemical processes on which the body operates.

Oxygen – a gaseous element essential for metabolism.

Oxytocin – a hormone secreted by the posterior pituitary gland; tends to raise the blood sugar level.

Pancreas – a large, glandular organ which secretes digestive enzymes into the intestines and insulin into the blood.

Parasympathetic nervous system – part of the autonomic nervous system which slows down body functions.

Pectoral breathing – breathing by expansion and contraction of the chest.

Pituitary gland – a small endocrine gland located in the midbrain. As it secretes hormones which regulate the function of all the other endocrine glands, it is considered to be the most important of the group.

291

Proteins – a group of complex organic compounds containing amino acids, the body's basic building blocks. In the body they are broken down to form carbohydrate or synthesized from carbohydrate.

Pulmonary circulation – blood circulation from the right ventricle of the heart to the lungs and back to the left atrium of the heart, for releasing carbon dioxide and absorbing oxygen.

Reticular formation – important nervous junction point in the brainstem; concerned mainly with the phenomena of arousal, alertness, sleep, emotional expression, regulation of posture, muscle tone and with involuntary visceral reactions.

Saline – salty.

Secretion – any substance which is released into the body by a gland or organ.

Septum – a thin muscular wall dividing two cavities.

Serous glands – the resting phase of mucus glands; they produce a thin, watery fluid.

Somatotrophic hormone – a growth hormone secreted by the anterior pituitary gland which stimulates skeletal and general body growth, increases protein synthesis, breaks down fat and raises the blood sugar level by increasing the synthesis of glucose while diminishing the rate of glucose consumption by the muscles.

Sphincter muscles – valves located at a number of points along the alimentary tract which control the movement of substances from one section of the digestive system to another.

Subcutaneous – located directly beneath the skin.

Sugars – a large group of carbohydrates which are used by the body for construction and maintenance of the cell structures and to provide energy for muscular activity.

Sympathetic nervous system – one half of the autonomic nervous system. The sympathetic nerves carry regulating impulses to most of the important bodily organs and when stimulated they raise the blood sugar level by increasing glycogenolysis and by stimulating adrenalin secretion.

Threshold – the lower limiting point which elicits a response when exceeded.

Thyroid gland – an important endocrine gland located in the throat; secretes thyroxin.

Thyrotrophic hormone – a hormone secreted by the anterior pituitary which stimulates the thyroid gland to secrete thyroxin.

Tissue – basic type of cell structure out of which organs and other parts of the body are built; used loosely to refer to subcutaneous and plain tissue separating the visceral organs.

Tissue fluid – a liquid which flows through all tissues in the body. It provides the cells with nourishment and removes their waste matter. It is supplied to and removed from the different areas by means of the tiny capillary endings of veins, arteries and lymphatics.

Trapezius muscles – muscles in the neck.

Vagus nerve – the most important parasympathetic nerve. It carries impulses from the brain to all of the organs in the visceral region. When stimulated, it tends to lower the blood sugar level by increasing insulin production.

References

Asthma: The Holistic Approach

[1] Ford, M., 'An allergist looks at asthma', *Mod. Med. Aust.*, Oct. 1979, 22(10):23–25.

[2] Lowen, A., *The Betrayal of the Body*, Collier, N.Y., 1967.

[3] Cohen, S.I., 'Psychological factors', in Clarke, T.J.H. and Godfrey, S., *Asthma*, Chapman and Hall, London, 1977.

[4] Groen, J.J., 'Psychosomatic Theory of Bronchial Asthma', Paper presented at the 4th Int. Congress of the Int. Coll. of Psychosom. Med., Kyoto, Japan, Sept. 1977.

[5] Crofton, J., Douglas, A., *Respiratory Diseases*, Oxford, Blackwell Scientific Pub., 1969, p.431.

[6] Selye, H., *The Stress of Life*, N.Y., McGraw Hill, 1976.

[7] Goyeche, J.R.M., 'Asthma: the yogic perspective, Part I: The somatopsychic imbalance in asthma: towards a holistic therapy', *F. Asthma Res.*, Apr. 1980, 17(3):111–121, p.111.

[8] Ibid, p.116.

[9] Goyeche, J.R.M., 'Asthma: the yogic perspective, Part II : Yoga therapy in the treatment of asthma', *E. Asthma*, 1982, 19(3):189–201, p.193.

Asthma: Holistic Therapy

[1] Alexander, A.B., Miklich, D.R. & Hershkoff, H., 'The immediate effect of systematic desensitization on peak expiratory flow rates in asthmatic children', *Psychosom. Med.*, 1972, 34:388–394.

[2] Alexander, A.B., 'Systematic desensitization and flow rates in asthmatic children: relationship to emotional participants and anxiety', *J. Psychosom. Res.*, 1972", 16:405–410.

[3] Alexander, A.B., Cropp, G.J.A. & Chai, H., 'Effects of relaxation training on pulmonary mechanics in children with asthma', *J. Apple. Behav. Anal.*, 1979, 12:27–35.

[4] Cooper, A.J., 'A case of bronchial asthma treated by behaviour therapy', *Behav. Res. Ther.*, 1964, 1:351–356.

[5] Davis, M.H., Sanders, D.R., Creer, T.L. & Chai, H., 'Relaxation training facilitated by biofeedback apparatus as a supplemental treatment in bronchial asthma", *J. Psychosom. Res.*, 1973, 17:121–128.

[6] Erskine, J.M. & Schonell, M.E., 'Relaxation therapy in bronchial asthma', *J. Psychosom. Res.*, 1979, 23:131–139.

[7] Feldman, G.M., 'The effects of biofeedback training on respiratory resistance of asthmatic children', *Psychosom. Med.*, 1976, 38(1) :27–34.

[8] Hock, R.A., et al., 'Medico-Psychological interventions in male asthmatic children: an evaluation of physiological change', *Psychosom. Med.*, May 1978, 40(3):210–215.

[9] Kahn, A.U., Staerk, M. & Bonk, C., 'Role of counter conditioning in the treatment of asthma', *J. of Psychosom. Res.*, 1974, 18:89.

[10] Kotses, H., et al., 'Operant reduction of frontalis EMG activity in the treatment of asthma in children', *J. Psychosom. Res.*, 1976, 20:453–459.

[11] Kotses, H., et al., 'Operant muscular relaxation and peak expiratory flow rate in asthmatic children', *J. Psychosom. Res.*, 1978, 22:17–23.

[12] Kotses, H., & Glaus, K.D., 'Facial muscle tension influences peak expiratory flow rate in normal and in asthmatic children (abst.)', *Biofeedback Self-Regulation*, 1978, 3:233.

[13] Miklich, D.R., et al., 'The clinical utility of behaviour therapy as an adjunctive treatment for asthma', *J. Allergy Clin. Immunol.*, 1977, 60(5):285–294.

[14] Moore, N., 'Behaviour therapy in bronchial asthma: a controlled study', *J. Psychosom. Res.* 1965, 9:257–276.

[15] Morwood, J.M.B., 'Relaxation by gramophone in asthma', *Practitioner*, 1953, 170:400–402.

295

[16] Philipp, R.L., Wilde, G.J.S., Day, J.H. 'Suggestion and relaxation in asthmatics', *J. Psychosom. Res.*, 1972, 16:193–204.

[17] Sargeant, H.G.S., & Yorkston, N.J., 'Verbal desensitization in the treatment of bronchial asthma', *Lancet*, 1969, 2:1321–1323.

[18] Scaeffer, G., & Freytag-Klinger, H., 'Objectifying the effect of autogenic training on disordered ventilation in bronchial asthma', *Psychiatr. Neurol. Med. Psychol.* (Leipz), 1975, 27(7):400–408.

[19] Scherr, M.S., Crawford, P.L. Serrgent, C.G. & Scherr, C.A., 'Effect of biofeedback techniques on chronic asthma in a summer camp environment', *Ann. Allergy*, 1975, 35:289–295.

[20] Smith, M.M., Colebatch, H.J.H. & Clarke, P.S., 'Increase and decrease in pulmonary resistance with hypnotic suggestion in asthma', *Am. Review of Resp. Dis.*, 1970, 102:236–242.

[21] Wilson, A.F., Hornsberger, R., Chiu, J.J. & Novey, H.S., 'TM and asthma', *Respiration* 1975, 32:74–80.

[22] Yorkston, N.J., et al., 'Verbal desensitization in bronchial asthma', *J. Psychosom. Res.*, 1974, 18:371–376.

[23] Yorkston, N.J. et al., 'Bronchial asthma: improved lung function after behaviour modification', *Psychosom Med.*, 1979, 20(5):325–331.

[24] Erskine-Milliss, J. & Schonell, M., 'Relaxation therapy in asthma: a critical review', *Psychosom. Med.*, Aug. 1981, 43(4):365–372.

[25] Goyeche, J.R.M., op.cit., 'Asthma: the yogic perspective, Part I', p. 118.

[26] Livingstone, J.L. & Gillespie, M., 'The value of breathing exercises in asthma', *The Lancet*, 1935, 705.

[27] Ibid.

[28] Barach, A.L., 'Breathing exercises in pulmonary emphysema and allied chronic respiratory disease', *Arch. Phys. Med. & Rehab.*, 1955, 36:379.

[29] Allan, W.B., 'Breathing exercises in pulmonary emphysema and allied chronic respiratory disease', *Arch. Phys. Med. & Rehab.*, 1955, 36:379.

[30] Erickson, D.J., 'Factors involved in posture', in: Krusen, F.H. (ed.), *Physical Medicine and Rehabilitation*, W.B. Saunders, Philadelphia, 1951.

[31] Fein, B., Cox, E.P. & Green, L.H., 'Respiratory and physical exercises in the treatment of bronchial asthma', *Ann. Allergy*, 1953, 11:275.

[32] 'Helping emphysema patients breathe more easily', *Your Family's Health*, Nov. 1983, p.31.

[33] Goyeche, J.R.M., 'Asthma: the yogic perspective, Part I', op.cit., p. 118.

[34] Katakov, A. Ju., 'Conscious hypoventilation at one breath per minute as a means of reducing metabolism', Abstract of the 1st conference on the applications of yoga in medicine, Praha, 1978.

[35] Tengshe, S.B., "Study of the effects of some pranayama practices of yoga on body functions", Ph.D. thesis submitted to All India Institute of Medical Sciences, New Delhi, June 1981.

[36] Kuvalyananda, S., Vinekar, S.L., *Yogic Therapy*, New Delhi, Ministry of Health, Government of India, 1963.

[37] Ibid.

[38] Stanescu, D.C., Nemery, B., Veriter, C. & Marechal, C., 'Pattern of breathing and ventilatory response to CO_2 in subjects practicing hatha yoga', *J. Appl. Physiol.*, 1981, 51(6):1625–1629.

[39] Miles, W.R., 'Oxygen consumption during three yoga-type breathing patterns', *J. Appl. Physiol.*, 1964, 19(1):75–82.

[40] Pratap, V., Berretini, W.H. & Smith, C., 'Arterial blood gases in pranayama practice', *Percept. and Motor skills*, 1978, 46:171–174.

[41] Schulte, H.J. & Abhyankar, V.V., 'Yogic breathing and psychologic strategy', *Arizona Medicine*, 1979, 36:681–683.

[42] 'Breathing cycle linked to hemispheric dominance', *Brain Mind Bulletin*, Jan. 3, 1983, 8(3):21–22.

[43] Ibid.

Diabetes Research

[1] Harris, J.A., 'Relaxation training as a stress reducing technique for persons with diabetes', *Dissertations Abst. Int.*, 1981, 41 (9):3573.

[2] *Diabetes*, 1979, 28(suppl. 1):107–110.

[3] 'Exercise therapy "rediscovered" for diabetes, but what does it do?', *JAMA*, Oct. 12, 1979, 242 (15):1591–1592.

[4] Ibid.

[5] Ibid.

[6] Pokordi, K, et al., 'Comparative studies on yoga, meditation and muscular exercise', Unpublished paper from Voluntary Health Services Medical Centre, Adyar, Madras.

[7] Shukla, H.S., et al, 'A clinical comparison of total gut irrigation with conventional bowel preparation for colorectal surgery', *J. Ind. Med. Assoc.*, May 1981, 76(10).

Clinical Trials

[1] Tandon, M.K., 'Adjunct treatment with yoga in chronic, severe airways obstruction', *Thorax*, 1978, 33:514–517.

[2] Divekar, M.V., *Yoga Awareness*, July 1971, 1(1).

[3] Sadhakas, X., *Yoga and Therapy*, Bombay, Examiner Press, 1977.

[4] Mehta, J.M. & Kurulkar, L.N., 'Yoga: The Key to Psychosomatics', paper read at the 4th Congress of the International College of Psychosomatic Medicine, Kyoto, Japan, Sept.5–9, 1977, published in the proceedings, p.141.

[5] Vorandani, N., Anandananda, Sw. Dharmveer, 'Diabetes and Yoga', paper presented to the First Scientific Seminar of the C.C.R.I.M.H. New Delhi, 1973.

[6] Goyeche, J.R.M., 'Asthma: the yogic perspective, Part 2; yoga therapy in the treatment of asthma', *J. of Asthma*, 1982, 19(3):189–201.

[7] Nagarathna, R. & Nagendra, H.R., 'Therapeutic Application of Yoga – A Report', Vivekananda Kendra, Report No. VKYTRC/001/KK/80.

[8] Bhole, M.V., 'Treatment of bronchial asthma by yogic methods', *Yoga Mimamsa*, 1967, 9(3):33.

[9] Rajyalaxmi Devi, S.R.Y., 'Therapeutic Modulation of Yoga on Diabetes Mellitus', unpublished manuscript, Indian Institute of Research in Yoga and Allied Science, Tirupathi, Andhra Pradesh.

[10] Srinivasin, T.M. & Meti, B.L., 'Management of Bronchial Asthma Through the Practice of Yogasana and Pranayama', unpublished manuscript, Indian Institute of Research in Yoga and Allied Sciences, Tirupathi, A.P.

[11] Singh, R., et al., 'Physiological and therapeutic studies on yoga', *The Yoga Review*, 1982, 2(4):185–209.

[12] Vahia, N.S., et al., 'Psychophysiological therapy based on the concept of Patanjali', *Am. J. Psychother*, 1973, 27:557.

[13] Rugmini, P.S. & Sinha, R.N., 'The effect of yoga therapy in diabetes mellitus', proc. seminar on Yoga, Science and Man, New Delhi, 1975.

How Yoga Works

[1] Udupa, K.N., Singh, R.H. & Shettiwar, R.M., 'Studies on physiological, endocrine and metabolic response to the practice of yoga in young normal volunteers', *J. Res. Ind. Med.*, 1971, 6(3):345–353.

[2] Udupa, K.N., Singh, R.H. & Shettiwar, R.M., 'Studies on physiological, endocrine and metabolic response to the practice of yoga', *J. Res. Ind. Med.*, 1972, 1:685.

[3] Udupa, K.N. & Singh, R.H., 'Scientific basis of yoga (letter)', *J. A. M. A.*, 1972 (June), 220:1365.

[4] Udupa, K.N., Singh, R.H. & Shettiwar, R.M., 'Physiological and biochemical studies on the effects of yogic and certain other exercises', *Ind. J. Med. Res.*, 1975, 63(4):620–624.

[5] Udupa, K.N., Singh, R.H. & Shettiwar, R.M., 'Studies on the effect of some yogic breathing exercises (pranayama) in normal persons', *Ind. J. Med. Res.*, 1975, 63(8):1062–1065.

[6] Udupa, K.N., et al., 'Comparative biochemical studies on meditation', *Ind. J. Med. Res.*, 1975, 63(12):1676–1679.

[7] Jevning, R., Wilson, A.F. & Smith, W.R., 'The TM technique, adrenocortical activity, and implications for stress', *Experientia*, 1978, 34(5):618–619.

[8] Michaels, R.R., Parra, J., McCann, D.S. & Vander, A.J., 'Renin, cortisol and aldosterone during TM', *Psychosom. Med.*, Feb. 1979, 41(1):50–54.

[9] Nayar, H.S., Sewamurthy, W., Joseph, N.T., Joseph, S. & Chohan, I. S., 'Effects of yogic practices on physiological and biochemical profile in man', Defense Institute of Physical and Allied Sciences, Delhi Cantt.

[10] Gopal, K.S., Natarajan, A. & Ramakrishnan, S., 'Biochemical studies in foreign volunteers practising hatha yoga', *J. Res. Ind. Med.*, 1974, 9(3):1–8.

Index of Practices

ABOUT THE AUTHOR

Dr Swami Shankardevananda
MBBS (Sydney), MSc (UNSW)

- Born in 1952 in Sydney, Australia, he graduated in medicine in 1977.
- While still a medical student he met his guru, Swami Satyananda Saraswati, in 1974, and was then able to blend alchemically the science of yoga and medicine into a unified system.
- He came to Bihar School of Yoga, Munger, India as Chief Coordinator of the IYFM Research Coordinating Centre in 1974.
- He received his MSc from the University of NSW in 1990 into the physiological effects of asana on the respiratory system.
- From 1990–2001 he coordinated the Sydney Yoga Therapy Research and Education Centre, combining a medical practice, complementary therapies and yoga classes.
- He now travels and teaches yoga around the world to support his guru's mission.
- He is also the author of: *The Effects of Yoga on Hypertension*, *The Practices of Yoga for the Digestive System* and *Amaroli*.

INTERNATIONAL YOGA FELLOWSHIP MOVEMENT (IYFM)

The IYFM is a charitable and philosophical movement founded by Swami Satyananda at Rajnandgaon in 1956 to disseminate the yogic tradition throughout the world. It forms the medium to convey the teachings of Swami Satyananda through its affiliated centres around the world. Swami Niranjanananda is the first Paramacharya of the International Yoga Fellowship Movement.

The IYFM provides guidance, systematized yoga training programs and sets teaching standards for all the affiliated yoga teachers, centres and ashrams. A Yoga Charter to consolidate and unify the humanitarian efforts of all sannyasin disciples, yoga teachers, spiritual seekers and well-wishers was introduced during the World Yoga Convention in 1993. Affiliation to this Yoga Charter enables the person to become a messenger of goodwill and peace in the world, through active involvement in various far-reaching yoga-related projects.

BIHAR SCHOOL OF YOGA (BSY)

The Bihar School of Yoga is a charitable and educational institution founded by Swami Satyananda at Munger in 1963, with the aim of imparting yogic training to all nationalities and to provide a focal point for a mass return to the ancient science of yoga. The Chief Patron of Bihar School of Yoga is Swami Niranjanananda. The original school, Sivanandashram, is the centre for the Munger locality. Ganga Darshan, the new school established in 1981, is situated on a historic hill with panoramic views of the river Ganges.

Yoga Health Management, Teacher Training, Sadhana, Kriya Yoga and other specialized courses are held throughout the year. BSY is also renowned for its sannyasa training and the initiation of female and foreign sannyasins.

BSY provides trained sannyasins and teachers for conducting yoga conventions, seminars and lectures tours around the world. It also contains a comprehensive research library and scientific research centre.

SIVANANDA MATH (SM)

Sivananda Math is a social and charitable institution founded by Swami Satyananda at Munger in 1984, in memory of his guru, Swami Sivananda Saraswati of Rishikesh. The Head Office is now situated at Rikhia in Deoghar district, Bihar. Swami Niranjanananda is the Chief Patron.

Sivananda Math aims to facilitate the growth of the weaker and underprivileged sections of society, especially rural communities. Its activities include: distribution of free scholarships, clothing, farm animals and food, the digging of tube-wells and construction of houses for the needy, assistance to farmers in ploughing and watering their fields. The Rikhia complex also houses a satellite dish system for providing global information to the villagers.

A medical clinic has been established for the provision of medical treatment, advice and education. Veterinary services are also provided. All services are provided free and universally to everyone, regardless of caste and creed.

YOGA RESEARCH FOUNDATION (YRF)

The Yoga Research Foundation is a scientific, research-oriented institution founded by Swami Satyananda at Munger in 1984. Swami Niranjanananda is the Chief Patron of the foundation.

YRF aims to provide an accurate assessment of the practices of different branches of yoga within a scientific framework, and to establish yoga as an essential science for the development of mankind. At present the foundation is working on projects in the areas of fundamental research and clinical research. It is also studying the effects of yoga on proficiency improvement in various social projects, e.g. army, prisoners, children. These projects are being carried out in affiliated centres worldwide.

YRF's future plans include literary, scriptural, medical and scientific investigations into other little-known aspects of yoga for physical health, mental well-being and spiritual upliftment.

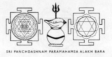

SRI PANCHDASHNAM PARAMAHAMSA ALAKH BARA

SRI PANCHDASHNAM PARAMAHAMSA
ALAKH BARA (PPAB)

Sri Panchdashnam Paramahamsa Alakh Bara was established in 1990 by Swami Satyananda at Rikhia, Deoghar, Bihar. It is a charitable, educational and non-profit making institution aiming to uphold and propagate the highest tradition of sannyasa, namely vairagya (dispassion), tyaga (renunciation) and tapasya (austerity). It propounds the tapovan style of living adopted by the rishis and munis of the vedic era and is intended only for sannyasins, renunciates, ascetics, tapasvis and paramahamsas. The Alakh Bara does not conduct any activities such as yoga teaching or preaching of any religion or religious concepts. The guidelines set down for the Alakh Bara are based on the classical vedic tradition of sadhana, tapasya and swadhyaya, or atma chintan.

Swami Satyananda, who resides permanently at the Alakh Bara, has performed the Panchagni Vidya and other vedic sadhanas, thus paving the way for future paramahamsas to uphold their tradition.

BIHAR YOGA BHARATI

BIHAR YOGA BHARATI (BYB)

Bihar Yoga Bharati was founded by Swami Niranjanananda in 1994 as an educational and charitable institution for advanced studies in yogic sciences. It is the culmination of the vision of Swami Sivananda and Swami Satyananda. BYB is the world's first government accredited university wholly devoted to teaching yoga. A comprehensive yogic education is imparted with provision to grant higher degrees in yogic studies such as MA, MSc, MPhil, DLitt, and PhD to the students. It offers a complete scientific and yogic education according to the needs of today, through the faculties of Yoga Philosophy, Yoga Psychology, Applied Yogic Science and Yogic Ecology.

Residential courses of four months to two years are conducted in a gurukul environment, so that along with yoga education, the spirit of seva (selfless service), samarpan (dedication) and karuna (compassion) for humankind is also imbibed by the students.

YOGA PUBLICATIONS TRUST (YPT)

Yoga Publications Trust (YPT) was established by Swami Niranjan-ananda in 2000. It is an organization devoted to the dissemination and promotion of yogic and allied knowledge – psychology (ancient and modern), ecology, medicine, vedic, upanishadic, tantric darshanas, philosophies (Eastern and Western), mysticism and spirituality – nationally and internationally through the distribution of books, magazines, audio and video cassettes and multimedia.

YPT is primarily concerned with publishing textbooks in the areas of yoga philosophy, psychology and applied yogic science, research materials, practice texts and the inspiring talks of eminent spiritual personalities and authors aimed at the upliftment of humanity by means of the eternal yogic knowledge, lifestyle and practice.